The Couple to Couple League International presents

The Art of Breastfeeding:

Empowering women to give their babies the best start

Written by Linda Kracht and Jackie Hilgert

The Art of Breastfeeding

Cover Design by Scott Bruno of b graphic design
Cover Photo by Ron Rack of Rack Photography

Cataloging data

Library of Congress Control Number: 2008929165

The Art of Breastfeeding
The Couple to Couple League
ISBN 978-0-926412-31-6

Published by
The Couple to Couple League International, Inc.
P.O. Box 111184
Cincinnati, OH 45211
U.S.A.

800-745-8252
www.ccli.org

Printed in the United States

10 9 8 7 6 5 4 3 2 1

Contents

Introduction

Prior to researching *The Art of Breastfeeding*, I thought I knew pretty much everything there was to know about the topic. I breastfed all seven of my children, and each brought unique needs, habits and challenges to the relationship. For thirty years, I also have been a teacher of Natural Family Planning for the Couple to Couple League, which has a long tradition of advocating breastfeeding. Certainly, I considered myself to be knowledgeable about breastfeeding.

However, my initial thought that writing this book ought to be a piece of cake vanished quickly as I realized I knew very little of the science behind breastfeeding, especially regarding how breastfeeding impacts women's health. What I learned in my research fully renewed my personal conviction and support for breastfeeding. Breastfeeding, in my opinion, should be front and center with regard to children and women's health issues.

Science has tried to capture the how and why of breastfeeding and much information has come to light that helps us be assured that breastfeeding is absolutely best for babies and mothers. Yet, as with other aspects of the human person, much of what makes breastfeeding the wonder that it is remains a mystery. There are intricacies and interdependencies that even scientists cannot explain; exactly how our human design allows us to feed and nurture our own is just a bit too complex for scientists to fully measure, explain or even replicate.

Thus, breastfeeding is more than mere science; breastfeeding is art. While researchers will always be interested in studying breastfeeding, perhaps in order to change how people can reap breastfeeding's many benefits without sacrifice — my belief is that breastfeeding is a gift God designed for mothers and babies, one that also benefits fathers and society as a whole.

In recent years, I've had the privilege of watching my grandchildren being breastfed. While their mothers breastfed under different circumstances — one worked full time while another breastfed twins *and* an older baby simultaneously — each of them made breastfeeding work because they were committed to doing what was best for their babies.

I believe that my adult children are able to embrace the art of breastfeeding because they observed me breastfeeding my babies, their siblings. They learned as youngsters the importance of sacrificing for the good of the children and now their efforts are a wonderful model for the art of breastfeeding. It is my hope this book touches other young mothers who will make the choice to practice the art of breastfeeding until their babies lead the weaning process.

More than simply understanding the underlying science, the art of breastfeeding is a developmental process that benefits both mother and baby. After reading this book, I'm confident you will be convinced that breastfeeding is best for all babies everywhere, including yours. I'm also confident as you practice the art of breastfeeding, you will learn its advantages for yourself, your husband, your family and society as well. It is, after all, part of God's design for the human family.

- Linda Kracht

Acknowledgements

I want to take a moment to thank my writing partner and editor, Jackie Hilgert; this book wouldn't have come together as it did without her efforts. We've given birth to this book as a team and upon completion, gained a greater understanding of the weaning process. It was gratifying to work with such a talented individual. I also need to thank Denise Cummings for her research assistance. Patricia Frey deserves credit for helping early in this book's development. Helping in our effort to offer clear and accurate information was Dr. Jack Burnham. Thank you for your careful review. Finally, a note of thanks to Giselle Alderson, Tom Bengtson and Ann Gundlach for the time they spent reviewing the manuscript.

A note about the cover: Shelly Schwartz of Cincinnati, Ohio, is breast-feeding six-week-old son, Abraham. During labor, Shelly experienced complications that necessitated an emergency Cesarean section; her complications worsened after childbirth and led to massive blood loss. Shelly required an emergency hysterectomy to save her life.

Because surgery left her weakened and apart from her newborn, Shelly was given little hope that breastfeeding would be successful. But with determination and under guidance of supportive medical professionals and lactation consultants, Shelly pumped colostrum every four hours while she recovered in intensive care. Once Shelly and Abraham were reunited: "little Abe has not missed a beat and has been an enthusiastic eater from the start."

Knowing the odds for successfully breastfeeding were stacked against them, Shelly considers their family very blessed. "Not all babies would have responded as well as he did," Shelly said.

After settling in at home, Shelly and her husband, Larry, have focused on developing the breastfeeding relationship. For his part, Abraham is thriving; he's gained, on average, one pound per week.

Shelly and Larry Schwartz are members of the Couple to Couple League.

Please note: For the purposes of this book, "baby" will always be referred to in the male gender.

CHAPTER ONE

The Art of Breastfeeding

Worthwhile human activity, whether it falls under the umbrella of science or the humanities, serves to advance society. Degrees in higher education also fall into one of two categories — science or art. It is easy to explain science: it is the pursuit of an objective truth. But what is this subjective thing we label art?

One may define art as an activity in which one demonstrates or hones a creative skill; one who devotes a lifetime to painting, for example, might be called *artist*. But art also references the principles or methods applied toward perfecting a craft; artists think creatively but also understand that skill is dependent upon being observant, planning ahead and practice. Art comes about through process.

It is in this vein that we consider breastfeeding to be an art. A woman who wants to breastfeed her child will need to learn new skills, techniques and principles in order to get the breastfeeding experience off to a good start. She will need to be observant. She will need to practice newly-acquired skills until they become second nature. But the process by which breastfeeding becomes "the art of breastfeeding" also requires a woman to continually learn — about herself, her baby, and about the challenges they each may encounter as they pursue breastfeeding through to its natural conclusion, which is when baby signals the desire to wean.

The decision to breastfeed a baby will impact the entire family and thus your curiosity about the worthiness of breastfeeding may have led you to this book. If so, welcome. Here you will discover that the art of breastfeeding not only gives your baby his best possible health and nutritional outcomes, but also that it respects baby's development and embraces the mother-baby, father-baby and husband-wife relationships. The art of breastfeeding is most certainly a worthwhile activity; when you learn and practice it, your efforts will help society advance just a bit further.

Breastfeeding: what will it mean for you?

Breastfeeding is a very unique human experience which greatly affects babies, mothers, fathers, and ultimately, society. Breastfeeding allows mothers to interact with babies and this interaction favors cognitive development. Women who breastfeed are more preoccupied with baby's development, are better able to sort out challenges that arise later, are able to respond instinctually to their babies, and have been shown to experience less postpartum depression. Thus, breastfeeding's benefits reach far beyond the basic fact that breast milk provides infants with unsurpassed nutrition.

For centuries, women from all cultures have provided their young with nature's consummate food — breast milk. For centuries, women have done this without the benefit of books, support networks, online resources or physician guidance. But society has changed greatly and so have the roles women have undertaken.

Chances are good that today's first-time mother juggles the affairs of the home with outside pursuits, which can include career, volunteer work, or education. It is likely she herself wasn't breastfed and hasn't had much exposure to others who've breastfed babies. Think about what your own exposure to this natural maternal biological response has been. If it is limited, you are not alone.

Because women are no longer naturally indoctrinated into a breastfeeding culture, the challenges to getting off to a good start and continuing down a sunny path to breastfeeding bliss can be significant. But they are not insurmountable.

This book addresses many of the challenges you may face in your desire to breastfeed your baby and it provides tactical solutions to help you overcome them. This book also addresses topics you may not have expected to encounter, such as societal notions that shift the longer you breastfeed *or* the evolution of your own attitudes toward breastfeeding.

You may choose, for instance, to commence breastfeeding for nutritional reasons but then find yourself continuing to breastfeed primarily for its nurturing capabilities. While nutrition and nurturing cannot be disassociated from one another, the emphasis can change several times throughout the breastfeeding experience and this shift should be expected. This text will prepare you for the changes that breastfeeding will bring about in you, your baby, your relationship with your spouse, your view of the world, and the world's view of you.

Carol Greer, who writes a column for the Couple to Couple League's *Family Foundations* magazine, described how she has seen other's attitudes toward breastfeeding shift: "In the estimation of many, nursing until Max was six weeks old made me a good mother; nursing to six months made me a very good mother; nursing to one year made me a hippy; nursing into his second year made me a fanatic." You, too, may discover that society both accepts and rejects your decision to breastfeed. This book will address these mixed messages so you can respond to them in your child's best interests.

You will read in these pages that continued breastfeeding, the term used here to describe breastfeeding that extends past baby's sixth month, may leave you feeling as if you are the only woman on earth who has given herself over to her baby and his needs. You may become discouraged by comments you overhear as you continue to breastfeed as baby approaches his first or even second birthday. When this happens, look to these pages for support. This book will give you the facts to counter popular notions, attitudes, and misinformation; hopefully it will feed your resolve to hone the skills you need to become an exceptional artist — one who feeds, nurtures and loves her baby in a mutually beneficial way.

Breastfeeding: a cultural norm?

Years of research have led to the discovery that breastfed babies have better overall health than formula-fed babies. Across the board, physicians and nutritionists agree that "breast is best" in providing for an infant's dietary needs, especially the needs of the pre-term infant. But the benefits of breastfeeding transcend simple nutrition. Breastfeeding benefits mother and baby in many ways. In fact, the benefits extend beyond mothers and babies to touch fathers and society as a whole; these benefits are classified as: **healthful, nutritional, immunological, developmental, social, psychological, economic** and **environmental**. You will find detailed information about these benefits in the next chapter.

The World Health Organization (WHO) recommends human milk for all infants. Its guidelines endorse exclusive breastfeeding (only breast milk) for all babies during the first six months of life, with breastfeeding continuing with complementary and supplementary solids to age twenty-four months or weaning. Recognizing the proven benefits of breastfeeding, the United States Department of Health and Human Services (HHS) adopted The 2010 Healthy People Objectives, which attempts to increase to at least 75 percent the proportion of mothers who exclusively or partially breastfeed their babies immediately after birth, and increase to at least 50 percent the proportion of women who continue breastfeeding until their babies are five to six months old. A further goal is to boost to at least 25 percent the proportion of babies who breastfeed to the age of twelve months. Currently in the United States, only 39 percent of babies are breastfeeding at age six months and only 21 percent of babies are breastfeeding at twelve months. At eighteen months, less than 7 percent of U.S. babies are still being breastfed.

In the United States, advocacy towards breastfeeding drops precipitously after a baby reaches six months of age. While enthusiasm and support for early and exclusive breastfeeding exists in all countries, the perceived importance for continued breastfeeding seems to exist only for developing countries, where hygiene, malnutrition rates, unsanitary drinking water, unavailability of food, and birth regulation are issues of concern. The pro-breastfeeding arguments seem pertinent only for women and babies living in poor countries, where parents' focus is often on getting their babies to survive beyond age five.

In the United States, by contrast, parents can rely on an established health care system to help them overcome the infant mortality concerns found throughout the Third World. This allows parents to shift focus toward helping their babies develop into strong adults — athletes and intellectuals — achievements not many will trace back to breastfeeding. Yet breastfed babies crawl and walk earlier than formula-fed babies. (Breastfed babies also eclipse their formula-fed counterparts in areas of emotional, immunologic, growth, psychological and overall health development.) So, continued breastfeeding offers a multitude of benefits in addition to meeting the basic needs of all parents, even those who live in developed countries with good health care, food aplenty, and excellent sanitation systems.

The HHS and WHO guidelines take into account what is best for baby. But the benefits of breastfeeding extend to mother, to father, and to society as a whole. These benefits will also be explored in the next chapter. But as you ponder what is best for your infant — and breast milk is clearly best — count on this text to give you information, skills, techniques, and tips to overcome any challenges that may come your way.

The process for learning an art

As part of learning the art of breastfeeding, you will learn to adapt your practices when situations arise that threaten your success. Things such as an inadequate milk supply, engorged breasts, sore nipples, fatigue, lowered libido, or pain during exercise may occasionally threaten your resolve to provide your baby with the consummate nutrition and bonding experience, one that cannot be replicated. Mothers who learn about the challenges they'll face in order to overcome them can perfect their breastfeeding technique and become more skilled and more artful over time and with the arrival of each new baby.

Be patient with yourself as you learn the techniques. Breastfeeding is not as easy to master as some may lead you to believe. (Give yourself and your baby time to learn and master the process.) Each baby brings his own temperament to the breast and this, along with shifting hormone levels, can make getting off to a good start challenging.

If you find you need more assistance or information than is available in this text, seek help from a breastfeeding resource, hospital hotline or certified lactation consultant. There is a list of resources to get you started at the back of this book.

Challenges aside, your innate love for your infant and your ability to nurture and care for him will instill confidence in your ability to provide for him throughout his life. This confidence will fuel your femininity, your sense of who you were created to be — a mother. In a study included in the book *Breastfeeding and Human Lactation*, breastfeeding was a main predictor of a woman's competence as a mother, competence being defined as the ability to make "independent child-care decisions, to find pleasure in parenthood, and to meet the demands of being a parent."

You will learn in these pages terms you may have not heard before: **exclusive breastfeeding** (no other foods or liquids given to an infant prior to the sixth month); **mixed breastfeeding** (formula or pumped breast milk given in addition to breastfeeding prior to the sixth month); **continued breastfeeding** (exclusive or mixed feeding that continues past the sixth month and/or introduction of complementary/supplementary foods); **complementary feeding** (adding nutrition after a breastfeeding session is finished when baby indicates continued hunger); and **supplementary feeding** (replacing breastfeeding calories with formula or solid foods). All of this information is presented in order to give you the knowledge you need to practice the art of breastfeeding and to practice this art to proficiency.

Until you deliver your first child and begin feeding him, the breastfeeding experience remains theoretical. Thus you may wonder: *What will it be like? How will I feel during breastfeeding? What sensations will I experience? What will be my comfort level, my attitude, or my acceptance of the breastfeeding experience?* The many effects, principles, experiences, and practices that become part of the breastfeeding experience are hard to measure. It is furthermore difficult to describe breastfeeding without talking in emotional terms.

How can you explain breastfeeding and not comment on how hypnotized you may become by gazing into your baby's eyes while breastfeeding him? How do you describe his little smirk or his excitement at latching onto the breast? What about the light that shines through his eyes as he gazes at you? Did you see his little feet kick, then immediately quiet? How happy did his delight at feeding at your breast make you feel? How can words describe these occurrences without reading like fantasy?

Likewise, how can a book on breastfeeding explain the superiority of breast milk using terms found in a physiology textbook without stripping the experience of all of its emotion?

This is also why we call breastfeeding an art.

There are procedures and techniques and plenty of science to be revealed that will support your decision to breastfeed, even to your most ardent detractors. But it is the unexplainable, indescribable aspects of breastfeeding that ultimately draw women to the art. It is mother's preoccupation, her innate desire to further her own child's development that allows her to overcome the times of pain, frustration, or perceived inconvenience, in order to breastfeed her child.

Motherhood and femininity look totally different when a mother surrenders herself first to God, then to her husband, then to her children. Confidence in a woman's ability to nurture and care for others fuels her sense of who she is. It defines her as feminine and thus through breastfeeding, through giving to her child, she gains a deeper understanding of how she was designed by the Creator.

Breastfeeding will provide you with the unique opportunity to nourish your baby with your own milk. In doing so, you will connect with your infant in a way that only you can. You have been equipped with breasts for the primary purpose of feeding your children. Through breastfeeding you will more fully experience your femininity.

CHAPTER TWO

Breast is Best — the Benefits

The phrase, "breast is best" was coined by an Austrian physician and researcher, Paul Gyorgy, M.D., in 1915. Gyorgy earned his medical degree and set out to research the cause of childhood rickets, which at the time was a leading cause of death among children. His research led him from the study of calcium, phosphorus and the chemistry of B vitamins (considered his major contribution to medicine) to investigations into yeast, egg white and, ultimately, milk.

Gyorgy discovered human milk far surpassed cow's milk when considering the components uniquely suited to the nutritional requirements of the human infant.[1] Furthermore, his study of animal milk instilled in him a staunch respect for the special properties contained in human milk, which transformed him into a breastfeeding advocate convicted of human milk's superiority in fulfilling the needs of infants. Gyrogy was adamant that manufactured formula never be allowed to replace human milk. Even though his colleagues supported the notion that science could improve upon nature, he didn't. When asked if formula could replace mother's milk, Gyorgy stated: "Breast is best; cow's milk is for calves."

The biochemistry of human milk is complex and its mysteries have been only partially unraveled. Scientists cannot capture the full essence of human milk because it is a living, changing substance. The composition of each mother's milk is unique to *her* and specially suited to the nutritional needs of *her* infant. A mother who delivers a pre-term infant, for example, will manufacture milk higher in protein and other immunological components than will a mother who delivers a full-term baby. Nature understands the nutritional needs of a preemie and provides for those needs. Furthermore, the composition of mother's milk changes during the breastfeeding continuum according to her baby's changing nutritional needs. Scientists understand this, yet they cannot explain it. Further, it confounds them as they attempt to isolate the quintessential sample of breast milk for the purpose of extracting its properties, and ultimately, replicating them.

(Breast milk cannot be duplicated or suitably replaced, despite claims made by many manufacturers of infant formula.) Formula is not the same as mother's milk and this substance, which has been artificially manufactured, packaged and shipped to a retailer for sale, cannot come close to human milk in meeting the nutritional needs of a developing human. (At the end of this chapter, you will find a hierarchy of infant feeding options; you may be surprised to learn how infant formula ranks among the many choices parents have at their disposal as they seek out the best way to feed their infant.)

Additionally, there is a discernable "breastfeeding edge" that your baby will enjoy once you learn, practice and become proficient in the art of breastfeeding. These advantages can be found through the following statistics:

> ▷ Three-fourths of baby's nutritional needs during his first year can be met solely through breast milk.

> ▷ A newborn has limited ability to produce his own antibodies to protect himself against disease.

> ▷ Breast milk contains antibodies, which enhance the infant antibody response.

> ▷ Breast milk protects against bacterial infection.

> ▷ The more breast milk an infant consumes, the greater his immunity to disease.

> ▷ Even when a mother gets sick, such as from a cold or the flu, her baby will be protected from infection through antigens passed along in breast milk.

It is important to remember that breastfeeding is about much more than simply providing good nutrition; breastfeeding has been called a broad spectrum medicine and its benefits reach babies, moms, dads, and all of society. Providing your baby with the best possible outcome is likely why you decided to seek knowledge in the art of breastfeeding. While nutrition is often touted as breastfeeding's big benefit, there are several others just as significant.

Health benefits

We think of primary disease prevention as any activity which keeps disease from taking hold in us. Secondary disease prevention would be an activity or action that reduces the severity of an illness, or ultimately cures us of it. Breastfeeding provides both types of disease protection. For infants born with little defense against disease, breastfeeding provides a solid arsenal with which the battle against viral and bacterial infections and allergies may be waged. There is limited but increasing evidence that continued breastfeeding is beneficial to child and mother; also, these benefits are not limited to full-term babies. Pre-term babies and babies with special needs who are breastfed reap health benefits that cannot be denied. Furthermore, these benefits are not limited to babies in developing countries; breastfeeding's benefits transcend socio-economic boundaries and borders.

Years of research reveal the overall health of breastfed babies is better than the overall health of their formula-fed counterparts. And mothers reap these health benefits, too. Each side is examined here separately.

Infant health advantages

Research in the United States, Canada, Europe and other developed countries provides strong evidence that breast milk decreases the incidence and/or severity of disease and allows for quicker recovery from distresses, including: diarrhea, lower respiratory infection, ear infection, blood poisoning, bacterial meningitis, botulism, urinary tract infection, and necrotizing enterocolitis (NEC), which is a bacterial affliction affecting premature and low birth weight infants. NEC is a very serious illness found more often among babies born weighing less than 1,500 grams (3.3 pounds) compared to near-term or term infants. There are further studies showing breastfeeding's protective effect against sudden infant death syndrome, asthma, pneumonia, diabetes, Crohn's disease, ulcerative colitis, lymphoma, leukemia, Hodgkin's disease, allergies and other chronic digestive maladies.[2]

The American Academy of Pediatrics reports that breastfed infants in the United States have a 21 percent lower infant mortality rate than formula-fed infants. Also, acute infections and hospitalizations are reduced for breastfed infants. Part of the reason may be because mother's milk is sterile and the perfect temperature for baby. Human milk contains a protein called lactoferrin, which inhibits the growth of E. coli; this protein is not found in manufactured infant formula.

Colostrum, or first milk, is known to help prevent respiratory syncytial virus (RSV), the most common reason infants are hospitalized. RSV is also a major contributor to high infant mortality.

Breast fed babies do not normally need supplemental iron during the first six months.[3] They receive and store iron from mother during the last two months of pregnancy and will absorb 60 percent of the iron present in breast milk. This is vastly greater than the iron absorption rate of formula-fed babies, which is roughly 4 percent. Baby does not begin to deplete iron stores until after age four to six months, which coincides with the start of complementary feeding and is the reason pediatricians call for iron-rich foods after six months.

Human milk contains sufficient amounts of all the necessary vitamins and minerals to meet the growing needs of infants, including fluoride. The American Academy of Pediatrics no longer recommends fluoride supplementation for breastfed infants.[4]

That said, an international debate is on-going regarding the need to supplement breastfed infants with vitamin D. A handful of reported cases of rickets (which causes soft, weak and malformed bones) have evoked a cautionary response from the U.S. Centers for Disease Control and the AAP to recommend breastfeeding mothers give 200 IU daily of liquid vitamin D to infants, older than two months of age. (Dark-skinned babies, or any baby with extremely limited sun exposure or whose mother does not eat meat, fish or dairy, are most at risk for developing rickets.)

Breastfeeding experts tie Vitamin D deficiency to lack of sunlight. Infants and older babies who are "adequately exposed to sunlight…and whose mothers consume adequate nutrients and are exposed to sunlight do not need vitamin D supplementation," according to the authors of *Breastfeeding and Human Lactation.*[6]

Exposure to sunlight naturally leads us to a concern for developing skin cancer. The question becomes: *how much sunlight is necessary?* The answer is complicated and controversial. The World Health Organization, the AAP, and the CDC recommend babies younger than age one not be exposed to direct sunlight, which creates a conflict to the human need for exposure to sunlight to produce Vitamin D.

Other research suggests that dark-skinned individuals require more sunlight exposure for adequate Vitamin D production than their fair-skinned brethren. Still other studies show skin pigment has no effect on Vitamin D production. Older studies from 1994 and 1985 recommended that infants receive thirty minutes of sunlight per week if wearing only a diaper and two hours per week when fully clothed, except for a hat.

"Skin is the human organ designed, in the presence of sunlight, both to manufacture Vitamin D in potentially vast quantities and to prevent the absorption of more than the body can safely use and store."[7] While some suggest breastfeeding mothers supplement with Vitamin D, others worry about the detrimental effect of overdosing. Vitamin D in too high a dosage (400 IU daily for infants) can be hazardous or potentially toxic. Parents need to be aware of the risk factors for Vitamin D deficiency and discuss them with their physician before supplementing Vitamin D.

Breast milk is especially crucial and linked to positive health outcomes with pre-term infants, who can struggle with heart, lung and circulatory abnormalities.

Continued breastfeeding contributes to a 52 percent reduction in development of celiac disease;[8] a similar observation has been reported with two types of childhood leukemia. Continued breastfeeding also reduces the severity and duration of ear infections in toddlers. Continued breastfeeding lessens long term adverse outcomes of diabetes during pregnancy even in the next generation. There is some evidence that continued breastfeeding after twenty-four months improves baby's overall health outcome compared to babies who have weaned from the breast. As mother continues to breastfeed, her milk changes, giving her older baby higher protective effects he'll need as he explores a germ-filled environment.

(Prior to age six months, infants lack the necessary digestive enzymes to completely digest complex proteins and starches found in ordinary foods.)The infant's intestine is susceptible to penetration by these proteins and starches, causing an immune response, which can lead to the development of allergies. (This is why exclusive breastfeeding is recommended for the first six months of baby's life and why you will want baby's single food source to be the optimum food source — breast milk.)

Remarkably, breastfed infants have higher blood cholesterol levels than do their formula-fed counterparts, due to the fact that human milk is high in cholesterol, an essential component of all membranes and required for growth. Yet, when breastfed infants reach adulthood, their cholesterol levels tend to be lower than their formula-fed counterparts. Animal studies suggest that by ingesting a high-cholesterol diet early, humans protect themselves from high cholesterol challenges later in life.

Continued breastfeeding hedges childhood obesity and the duration of breastfeeding corresponds with the protective effect. Breastfeeding also impacts how baby's mouth, jaw, palate and teeth develop. Breastfeeding helps maintain good occlusion while developing the palate into a well-rounded and full U-shaped arch. The action of baby's tongue pushing against the roof of the mouth also raises the floor of the nasal cavity, increasing nasal space between the bridge of the nose and the sinuses, reducing snoring and obstructive sleep apnea.[9]

The benefits of breastfeeding stay with people for a lifetime. There is limited evidence showing that adults continue to enjoy the health benefits of having been breastfed — they report fewer incidences of high blood pressure, heart disease, obesity, diabetes, hardening of the arteries, and celiac disease.

Maternal health advantages

While a woman's postpartum health issues are multi-faceted, evidence points to her enjoying reasonable health benefits while breastfeeding, including emotional and psychological advantages. One of these relates directly to the effect breastfeeding has on her body immediately after childbirth. A newborn's suck on the breast increases levels of the hormones oxytocin and prolactin, resulting in accelerated shrinking of the uterus, which reduces postpartum bleeding and lowers the risk of developing anemia. All of these benefits facilitate postpartum recovery. Oxytocin has been called the "hormone of love" because it has a relationship with orgasm, birth, breastfeeding and bonding.

Beyond the postpartum benefits breastfeeding women enjoy, there are physiological changes underway that could have far-reaching effects. One such benefit is the increased heart function during lactation, which results in more oxygen flowing through her body and a heart that beats more efficiently.

Also, there is increased blood flow to the mammary glands which both increases milk production and helps nourish breast cells.[10] It seems logical that a fully developed and well-nourished breast stands better protected against cancer-causing agents; does this explain why there's a link between breastfeeding and a reduced risk for developing premenopausal breast cancer? Interruption of ovulation and/or modifying the pituitary and ovarian hormones during breastfeeding have been assigned as reasons for a decrease in premenopausal breast cancer.[11] A study published in *The New England Journal of Medicine* advised: "If all pregnant mothers breastfeed for twenty-four months or longer, breast cancer could be reduced by 25 percent or more, for women who lactate at an early age."[12]

Breastfeeding also is linked to a reduced risk for developing uterine, endometrial and ovarian cancers. Researchers have found lactation leads to improved bone re-mineralization, thus breastfeeding women retain calcium better than non-breastfeeding women. This manifests itself in a reduced risk for later-in-life hip fractures and osteoporosis.

Breastfeeding also improves the functions of the gastrointestinal systems in women. Lactating women produce many hormones, some which aid digestion, promote insulin release, and stimulate metabolism, which facilitates weight loss. One study found that breastfeeding mothers lost significantly more weight than non breastfeeding mothers by six months postpartum.[13] The weight loss was positively associated with a reduction in body mass index. Breastfeeding mothers also have a lower incidence of obesity later in life. Breastfeeding offers a protective effect against glucose intolerance, an important benefit in a society where diabetes has become a public health crisis.

Also, exclusive breastfeeding normally postpones ovarian function for months following childbirth, freeing mother from closely-spaced pregnancies so that she may attend to herself, her baby and her family, while also allowing her to rebuild her own energy and strength. The temporary cessation of ovarian function and menstruation due to breastfeeding, called lactational amenorrhea, gives couples a natural baby spacing ability. (Lactational amenorrhea is discussed in chapter seven.)

Research has shown that women who are exposed to less estrogen over their lifetime (due to pregnancy, breastfeeding, and a later start of menses during puberty) are more protected against breast, uterine and ovarian cancers. Thus, while women breastfeed for baby's sake, many physical and emotional benefits extend to her as well.

Immunological benefits

We all know that anxiety, stress, and anger can negatively affect our immune systems. Hormones are typically involved in the rise and fall of depression, anxiety and anger. Women engrossed in the art of breastfeeding will discover that breastfeeding hormones can squelch negative moods and have a positive effect on the immune system. But breastfeeding has a far greater impact on baby's immune system.

Baby has an immature immune system until he reaches age twenty-four months. He receives some immunity from the placenta during the birthing process, but he receives the most valuable living immunities on an ongoing basis from mother's milk; this not only offers protections but allows him time to develop his own immune system. Mother's milk contains immunologic agents which act against viruses, bacteria and parasites. Breastfeeding provides both primary and secondary protection against these afflictions. If you deprive an infant of mother's milk, you remove a vital component to his immune system, leaving him vulnerable to a host of trouble from viruses, bacteria, and parasites.

Children who are breastfed exclusively have fewer illnesses than those who never breastfeed. While protection against infection is strongest during the first months of life, studies show immune protection continues even after breastfeeding ceases. The longer baby breastfeeds, the stronger the protective effect.

Mother's milk is sterile, species-specific and the perfect temperature for baby. Breast milk is a living substance adapting daily and even hourly to baby's age and needs. His mother's milk is always appropriate whether he is delivered at term or early.

Preterm infants are born with immature intestinal tracts and lower antioxidant capacities. They also are often exposed to oxidative stressors, such as mechanical ventilators, blood transfusions, IV drips, and an environment ripe for infection. All of these factors work against baby as he struggles to survive. Common disorders which may result include: lung disease, NEC, retinopathy (eye disease), and brain bleeds. By ingesting human milk, antioxidant capacities rapidly increase in preterm infants. Researchers know that human milk has better antioxidant protection than manufactured infant formula.

Breast milk contains high concentrations of immune globulin A (IgA), which fights infection. IgA is the most biologically active of all the immunoglobulins present in breast milk. IgA is available only through mother's milk; babies cannot produce it until about six months of age. Furthermore, IgA is not present in manufactured infant formula.

The total amount of key ingredients, such as infection fighting immunoglobulins, remains relatively constant throughout lactation. These concentrations increase as total breast milk volume decreases. In other words, as baby begins to wean, he still receives the same infection protection as when he was exclusively breastfed even though he is consuming less milk.

Through breast milk, babies receive protection from illnesses and the environment to which mother is exposed. Even if mother is sick with a cold, the flu, or diarrhea, her breast milk will produce antibodies to these illnesses, offering baby protection. This is why breastfed babies have fewer hospitalizations and more protection against the severity and incidence of chronic and acute infectious diseases.

The list of immunological protections can go on and on. Suffice it to say, breast milk, with its anti-infective properties, is key to providing the most favorable health outcome for your baby.

Nutritional benefits

Mother's milk plays multiple roles; it offers immunological protections and nutritional benefits. Breast milk is the perfect infant nutrition; it is sterile, easy to digest, and will satisfy both hunger and sucking needs. Breast milk contains more than two hundred known nutritional and functional components allowing baby to thrive on this single food source for his first six months of life. By contrast, manufactured infant formula contains roughly half of these known components.

Breast milk is good food — it is good for all babies, regardless of age. Breast milk contains key components vital to brain growth, vitamins, appropriate calories and immunological properties second to none. The fat content of breast milk depends upon many variables: mother's weight gain during pregnancy, the time between feedings, the degree of breast fullness, and the duration of each feeding at one particular breast. Fat content is important for baby to gain weight; it also eases digestion. The fat content in breast milk decreases after five or six months coinciding with the need for complementary foods.

Fat content may be four to five times greater in **hind milk** (the milk present at the end of a breastfeeding session) than in **fore milk** (the milk present at the beginning of a session), making it important that baby not be removed from the breast prematurely. If he is, he may not receive adequate nutrients, fats, proteins and calories and may become fussy or colicky. Remember that the fat received later in a feeding provides the most concentrated source of energy for your baby.[14]

In fact, "about twelve percent of baby's calories are consumed between eleven and sixteen minutes after beginning breastfeeding," according to *Counseling the Nursing Mother*. Furthermore, hind milk fat takes longer to digest than fore milk; fore milk is higher than hind milk in carbohydrates and sugars. Therefore infants who take in enough hind milk are more satisfied and less likely to act colicky or need to go to the breast as often. Hind milk is nature's mechanism for controlling baby's appetite — as he intakes milk fat he will begin to feel fuller and more satisfied.

Sometimes first-time breastfeeding mothers worry they do not have enough milk because their baby wants to breastfeed often — even hourly. But the frequency with which a baby feeds is related more to the digestibility of his mother's milk than the quantity of her milk. The average baby will digest breast milk in an hour and a half. Contrast this with the time it takes for a baby to digest manufactured infant formula — two and one half hours — and you will understand why baby wants to nurse so frequently. Mothers who understand that breast milk is much easier to digest than manufactured infant formula can begin to relax as they learn frequent breastfeeding is normal.

Another benefit to breast milk's digestibility is that it does not place metabolic stress on baby's immature organs, especially the kidneys. Cow's milk is higher in total protein and casein, making it less digestible and more stressful to immature kidneys. Human milk provides lipids and enzymes, which promote efficient digestion and utilization of nutrients. It is fully digestible and absorbable. A breastfed baby's stool will be softer and less-offensive smelling, too, because it contains a fatty acid soap, a byproduct of digesting breast milk.

Mothers concerned about whether they have enough milk need to look for more "telling" clues to whether baby is ingesting enough milk, such as weight gain and wet diapers. It is important to understand breastfeeding norms regarding feeding frequency because they differ considerably from formula-feeding norms.

Some also believe that breastfed babies need extra water or fluid supplements, especially in hot, dry climates. This notion is not supported by scientific data or studies. Anthropologists studying early civilizations, including those living in hot, dry climates, note women were able to nourish and hydrate infants exclusively through breastfeeding.

Research indicates breast milk is roughly 90 percent water, providing baby with enough fluid in the early months to satisfy his requirements. Furthermore, the water in breast milk provides baby a temperature regulating mechanism. Newborns lose approximately one fourth of their body heat due to evaporation of water from the lungs and skin.

Mother should be able to rely exclusively on breastfeeding to fully nourish her baby at least until he is old enough to eat complementary foods, roughly at age six months. But breastfeeding supplies 75 percent of baby's caloric requirements until he reaches the age of twelve months. Therefore, complementary foods ought to be low in calorie and high in nutrition to insure baby is not overfed.

Because breast milk's fat content declines over time, continued breastfeeding offers older babies the opportunity to receive optimal nutrition with adequate calories; babies who are continually fed manufactured formula may exceed their calorie requirements by as much as 35 percent once solid foods are worked into their diets. Overfeeding leads to lower metabolic rates in infants and more stress on developing organs; it also can lead to obesity.

While breastfed babies under age six months may appear chunkier than their formula-fed counterparts, due to the high fat content in breast milk, formula-fed babies will eclipse breastfed babies in overall weight after six months of age. In a study cited in the text *Breastfeeding and*

Human Lactation, by eight months of age, breastfed infants will have consumed thirty thousand fewer calories than formula-fed infants.[15] Further research involving more than one hundred thousand children shows an inverse linear association between the duration of breastfeeding and the risk of childhood obesity: the longer baby breastfeeds, the lower his risk of a lifetime struggle with weight and all its related issues.

Breast milk is not a static fluid but a living secretion of the mammary gland; its composition is constantly changing. As concentrations of protein, fat, carbohydrates, minerals and cells differ, its physical properties change. The impact of these changes, and their resulting effect on the infant's intestinal system, is only beginning to be understood.

Developmental benefits

There are observable differences between breastfed infants and their formula-fed counterparts in the areas of physical and cognitive development. Growth charts used in the United States until the year 2000 led to confusion about the growth of breastfed infants. These charts utilized curves derived from an infant population whose majority was formula fed. The Centers for Disease Control subsequently revised these growth charts; however, they still poorly reflect the appropriate growth curve of the breastfed baby.

The World Health Organization has developed a new set of growth charts based on healthy, breastfed infants' weight, height, length, and head circumference (see Figures 2-1 and 2-2, page 22). Growth charts, however, can create anxiety for parents when they do not understand, or have not been adequately informed, of their purpose. Growth charts are meant to insure a baby follows his own appropriate development; it is not meant to compare one infant's development to another's. Many a breastfeeding mother has been given inappropriate or misguided advice on her baby's development because of how his growth was measured and plotted on a growth chart.

You may have heard that breastfed babies generally crawl and walk sooner than formula-fed infants. It is true! But the developmental edge — or breastfeeding edge — does not end there (see Figures 2-3, page 23).

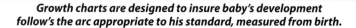

Growth charts are designed to insure baby's development follow's the arc appropriate to his standard, measured from birth.

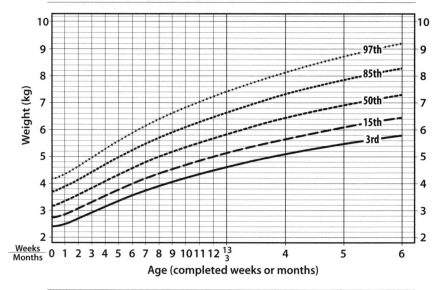

FIGURE 2-1. Weight-for-age Girls (Birth to 6 months — percentiles).
Source: WHO Child Growth Standards, http://www.who.int/childgrowth/standards/chts_girls_p.pdf.

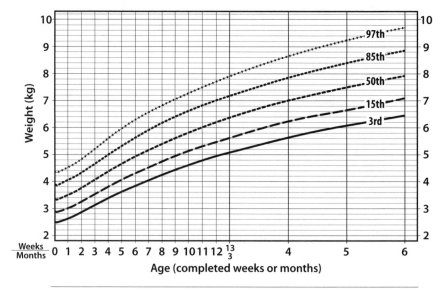

FIGURE 2-2. Weight-for-age Boys (Birth to 6 months — percentiles).
Source: WHO Child Growth Standards, http://www.who.int/childgrowth/standards/chts_boys_p.pdf.

If there was a nutrition label attached to a woman's breast, water would be listed as the number one ingredient in breast milk, followed next by lipids. (Lipids and triglycerides compose 5 percent of human milk.) There are 160 long-chain polyunsaturated fatty acids alone in human milk, which are crucial to brain and visual development. For this reason, breast milk fats continue to generate intense interest among lactation experts. The composition of breast milk and its developmental qualities also have captured the attention of formula manufacturers, who often make the claim that their product is "most like mother's milk." However, although manufacturers may attempt to replicate naturally-synthesized fats by using vegetable and animal sources, they cannot replicate or duplicate *human* essential fatty acids or long-chain polyunsaturated fatty acids. Where are all these lipids at work inside of baby? With his brain development, of course!

Several studies that measured the intelligence quotient (IQ) of breast-fed infants compared to formula-fed infants (using the Bayley Mental

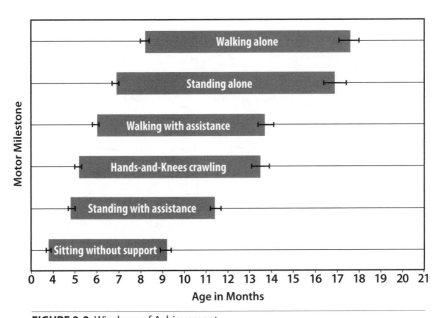

FIGURE 2-3. Windows of Achievement
Source: WHO Child Growth Standards, http://www.who.int/childgrowth/standards/cht_windows.pdf.

Development Index) showed breastfed infants had, on average, a 3.18 higher IQ than formula-fed babies.[16] While three points may seem insignificant, the advantage is measurable. Consider a person who has an IQ of 103 versus 100. This jump in IQ would elevate an individual from the fiftieth percentile of the population to the fifty-eighth percentile of the population. It also would be associated with higher educational achievement, occupational achievement and social adjustment.[17] The jump is more substantial with infants of low- and very-low birth weight, manifesting in reduced special education services necessary to educate many of these children. In this way, breastfeeding brings about societal benefits, too.

Furthermore, a report published in the May 2008 *Archives of General Psychiatry*, reports how breastfed infants fared in a study conducted in Belarus. Researchers randomly assigned 7,108 infants to exclusive breastfeeding and another 6,781 infants to breastfeeding plus other foods. When the children were six-and-a-half years old, they were given standard IQ tests. The children who were exclusively breastfed scored, on average, 7.5 points higher in verbal intelligence, 2.9 points higher in nonverbal intelligence, and 5.9 points higher in overall intelligence.

Cognitive benefits increase with continued breastfeeding. The results outlined above were found to be directly proportional to the amount of breast milk ingested in relation to the weight of the baby. Some suggest the cognitive edge is due in part to the improved mother-infant interaction during breastfeeding. Clearly, breastfeeding maximizes baby's early potential, including his cognitive development.

Furthermore, human milk is flavorful and variable, depending upon mother's diet; as a result, studies show breastfeeding babies develop more fully their sense of taste and smell. Products such as garlic, mint, vanilla and cheese alter the taste and smell of breast milk. This isn't necessarily a negative; babies enjoy variety. Studies reveal a baby will stay at the breast longer when the breast milk smells of garlic. If mothers vary their diet frequently, baby will adjust to new tastes and develop into a less-picky eater, according to one study.[18]

Also, if mother is a healthy eater during pregnancy and lactation, weaned babies will be more inclined to accept healthy foods when given a choice; this can be an important benefit as you teach your child to adopt a healthier lifestyle.[17] One should not discount the importance of early exposures when examining adult food preferences. Breastfeeding babies self-regulate their food intake, a significant behavioral benefit as they grow into adulthood and face unlimited food choices, many of them unhealthy. Early exposure to a healthier food choice may improve acceptance of healthy foods after weaning.

One more advantage to breastfeeding was reported in a Robert Wood Johnson University Hospital article published in July 2006 which linked formula-feeding to the increased incidence of bed-wetting, likely caused by delayed neurodevelopment. Exclusive breastfeeding was linked to a lower likelihood of bed-wetting during childhood while breastfeeding supplemented with formula did not offer the same benefit of reduced bed-wetting rates.

Psychological benefits

To many, the major benefit to breastfeeding is the emotional well-being it instills in both mother and child. A breastfeeding mother will slow down and give her child undivided attention many times each day. She'll look into his eyes. She'll talk to him. She'll touch him and he will touch her. They connect in a unique way. This connection facilitated through breastfeeding provides baby with comfort — physically, emotionally and psychologically. It also contributes to his cognitive development.

In her book *Cultural Breastfeeding*, anthropologist Kathyrn Dettwyler draws a beautiful picture of the breastfeeding relationship: "The distance from the infant to mother is perfect for the breastfeeding newborn to visualize her face. The closeness against the chest wall allows him to experience the maternal heartbeat, a familiar sound. The warmth of the lactating breast replaces the familiar warmth of the uterus."

Breastfeeding builds a bond between mother and child and their closeness strengthens throughout the breastfeeding relationship; it is not easily lost once breastfeeding ceases. Some have called mothers and babies engaged in breastfeeding "mutual caregivers." Baby receives care yet he also allows mother to reap important benefits, such as an increased con-

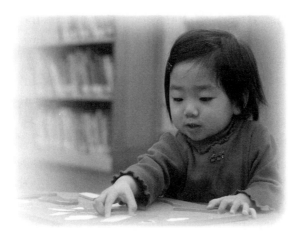

fidence in her ability to make independent child-care decisions, and the ability to meet the demands of mothering while simultaneously enjoying motherhood. Babies rely on cradling, touch, smell, sounds, and movement to feel secure — even to survive. As babies age and gain independence, they develop curiosity and trust in the world around them. This is positive emotional growth stemming from the attachment that is fundamental to the art of breastfeeding. Early dependence and attachment fosters later independence. Yet the bond endures. Even children between the ages of fifteen and eighteen who were breastfed tend to remain appropriately attached to their parents.

The process of becoming an individual begins when baby realizes he is separate from his mother. The process unfolds slowly. Between eighteen months and thirty-six months, an older baby still very much needs his mother in order to feel secure. But, as he broadens his ability to recognize his existence separate from his mother, he will begin to tolerate brief periods of separation and his world will expand to include his father — also an important figure in his development. Together, mother and father hold baby's best interests in perfect balance with their own; no one is left behind in a loving family. Each person's needs are considered and accommodated to the best of their ability. Needs are placed above self; mother and father essentially die to self in order to raise their children.

Maria Montessori in her book *The Absorbent Mind*, writes: "Localized states of maturity must first be established and the effort to force the child's natural development can only do harm. It is nature that directs."

Family life gets busier as baby grows; often, a busy older baby must compete for his mother's attention. Here again, there is value in continuing the breastfeeding relationship. Breastfeeding forces both mother and older baby to slow down. Through breastfeeding, an older baby gets the undivided attention he craves from his mother and she can use the time to relax, unwind, and focus on him.

Breastfeeding also can offer relief to babies who experience chronic pain or even sudden pain, such as from a vaccination or fall. You may think the soothing effect found in breastfeeding is the result of him being distracted, but there are explanations rooted in science. Hormones released by suckling and absorption of milk fat induce relaxation and pain relief. Also the sweet milk stimulates a narcotic-like effect in the brain, decreasing the perception of pain. Finally, the skin-to-skin contact reduces stress and blood pressure, and helps stabilize body temperature and breathing rates.[20]

Continued breastfeeding also increases a child's coping mechanism during stressful times. It further reduces his need to replace mother with an inanimate comfort object such as a blanket or toy. Psychological benefits to baby continue even after breastfeeding ceases.

For mother, the soothing effect of oxytocin released during breastfeeding has been noted by researchers to lead to a significantly lower incidence of child mistreatment or child neglect. Although research on the mechanisms of relaxation and analgesia has focused on newborns, these calming effects work synergistically; many mothers report these for the duration of breastfeeding.

Breastfeeding confers other psychological benefits to women. Breastfeeding hormones help mothers avoid anger or negative moods, help them sleep better, and reduce stress which may result in feeling less depressed, a benefit enjoyed also by their babies.

For some women, however, depression is real; for these women, breastfeeding can be a helpful way to manage depression. A woman who needs medications to manage her depression is cautioned to closely consult with her physician as she pursues breastfeeding. By communicating her breastfeeding goals, her physician can help her avoid ingesting antidepressants that could harm her baby or reduce her milk supply. A physician committed to helping a woman succeed with breastfeeding despite her depression will acknowledge that breastfeeding can be part of her treatment plan.

Medications aside, maternal depression has shown to produce abnormal brain patterns only in non-breastfeeding babies. Breastfeeding offers a protective effect from abnormal brain patterns in babies even if mother is depressed, another important benefit enjoyed through breastfeeding.

Economic benefits

Pro-breastfeeding arguments often have focused on Third World countries, where women do not have access to adequate food, water, sanitation, and medical care. In such circumstances, infants indeed benefit from exclusive and continued breastfeeding. In fact, the World Health Organization recommends babies breastfeed to age twenty-four months or longer. Yet economically disadvantaged families are not limited to the Third World. The U.S. government historically has responded to its own poor families' nutritional needs through programs such as Women, Infants and Children (WIC), which distributes a half a billion dollars worth of manufactured infant formula each year. The consequences of this policy are far-reaching and some argue it drives down acceptance and adoption of the healthier practice of exclusive breastfeeding. A policy that distributes free formula to disadvantaged families runs in direct opposition to The 2010 Healthy People Initiative, which calls for an increase in breastfeeding rates. It can be difficult for some women to take the initiative to breastfeed when free formula is dropped in their laps.

Considering the health and immunologic benefits outlined above, if women met the breastfeeding goals of The 2010 Healthy People Initiative, more than one billion dollars could be saved annually in health care costs, more than two-hundred million dollars annually in reduced incidence of RSV cases alone.

A change in policy, however, may not be easy to achieve, considering formula manufacturers are part of a two-billion- to three-billion-dollar industry, which provides jobs and tax revenues.

A 1997 study by Holy and Weimer[21] found breastfed babies had fewer hospital admissions and their total medical costs averaged less than formula-fed infants.

Closer to home, purchasing manufactured infant formula can make a significant impact on a family budget, costing between nine hundred dollars and twelve hundred dollars per year, (using 2007 prices) based on using less-expensive powdered formula. When you factor in that formula-fed infants do not reap the health benefits inherent from consuming human milk (which may result in more frequent and more severe health problems), the economic savings from breastfeeding can be staggering, some have estimated as high as three-and-a-half billion dollars annually.

Families that struggle to pay for manufactured formula may dilute it in order to make it last longer, may introduce inappropriate supplementary foods such as sugared fruit drinks, or may abandon formula in favor of less expensive cow's milk. In extreme circumstances, the cost of formula use may be such a significant drain on a family budget that other family members may be undernourished leading to further healthcare, social and developmental consequences.

A study conducted with employees of a Los Angeles public works department found support for breastfeeding at the workplace reaped economic benefits through reduced absenteeism, improved recruiting and retention rates, increased productivity, reduced infant health care expenses and reduced maternal stress.

The decision to breastfeed has economic consequences for families, communities and society as a whole. Because human milk is vastly superior to manufactured infant formula, the economic consequences of breastfeeding versus not breastfeeding extend far beyond a family's monthly grocery bill. Added costs include out of pocket healthcare, increased insurance premiums, reduced wages due to caring for sick babies, waste, and increased time shopping for and cleaning bottle-feeding supplies.

It does not take any time to prepare to breastfeed and the time spent breastfeeding is your best investment in your baby's emotional health and physical well-being. The enjoyable art of breastfeeding truly creates a breastfeeding edge!

Environmental benefits

In contemporary terminology, breastfeeding is "green" or "organic." Breast milk is readily-available, the perfect temperature and environmentally-friendly; its manufacture does not place additional burden on natural resources (paper, oil, aluminum), it does not require packaging, storage, transportation, or refrigeration. Its package will never end up in a landfill!

What is more, breast milk will never be recalled due to contamination. The environmental advantages of breastfeeding benefit families indirectly and society directly.

Social benefits

The pattern of the whole — breastfeeding is best for mother, baby, father, society — is found in each of its parts: nutritional, healthful, developmental, immunological, pyschological, economic and environmental. All of the benefits reaped by mothers and babies who breastfeed, described above, combine to create its social benefit. The social benefit, in turn, benefits mothers, babies, fathers and all of society. For instance, healthier babies decrease the burden on society's healthcare system, cognitive benefits ease the burden on society's educational system, and immunological benefits impact the corporate world by reducing absenteeism, significant especially for small companies.

Sadly, because breastfeeding has lost its standing as a social norm, women who choose to give their babies the best possible outcome through breastfeeding may encounter negative social consequences. These include a mother feeling excluded, isolated, disconnected and vulnerable. Further, women may find they are openly criticized by strangers, friends, or even family members who do not understand or support the decision to practice the art of breastfeeding — especially as their babies grow older. This can cause some women to retreat, engaging in **closeted breastfeeding,** behavior that further exacerbates the sense of isolation and vulnerability.

When mothers hide their breastfeeding practice from others, it becomes virtually impossible to reverse society's antagonism toward breastfeeding no matter the age of the baby. Hiding also hinders women's ability to accept their femininity and breastfeeding's role in advancing society, which can lead to prematurely abandoning the practice. When women buckle under negative pressure, weaning isn't baby-led but becomes socially coerced. Women who feel they must breastfeed hidden away in a public restroom rather than doing so modestly in a comfortable, open environment, deny their own and their babies' dignity along with all the proven benefits of natural feeding. This denial gives further credence to society's notion that women's breasts are sexual objects, not organs created primarily for the purpose of nurturing and feeding children. (The repercussions of the American culture's over-sexualization of women's breasts is examined in chapter five.)

It is worth noting here that mothers who practice continued breastfeeding report more positives than negatives about their experience — these are women who have mastered the art of breastfeeding.

You may choose initially to breastfeed your baby for health and nutritional benefits. Down the road, you may find your original reasons become less important as you continue; this is when the emotional benefits eclipse the nutritional benefits. If you can find support for your decision to continue breastfeeding from your spouse and from other mothers, you will further develop your confidence, which will become an important buffer for you against the criticism of others. Even if these criticisms continue and cause you negative feelings, you will find they have little impact on your resolve to breastfeed. When this occurs, congratulations are in order. You, too, have mastered the art of breastfeeding! What's more, your baby will have mastered the art, too, for he does not want to give it up until he is developmentally ready — no matter what others say.

Infant feeding options

The hierarchy of feeding allows families to make informed decisions that best match a particular infant's needs. The hierarchy lists infant food choices from the best available option to the least beneficial option. This information is compiled from the World Health Organization Hierarchy of Feeding Choices, among other sources, and is provided so that you will understand that infant feeding choices involve more than simply choosing between breastfeeding and formula-feeding.

Hierarchy of infant feeding

1. **Breast milk provided by exclusive breastfeeding.** Maximum benefits include: immunologically active, bonding, emotional, nutritional (a living substance), disease prevention, easily digestible, and adapts to a growing baby's needs. Composition matches baby's daily demand and chronological age, and contains more than 200 components.

2. **Fresh breast milk, pumped and immediately fed to baby.** Benefits include most of those listed above. Problems include limited handling, possible contamination during collection and unsanitary equipment. Can diminish milk supply if collection occurs too infrequently.

3. **Fresh pre-term breast milk, pumped and immediately fed to baby.** Considerations the same as above, but baby may need supplemental calcium and vitamin D.

4. **Donated fresh pre-term breast milk.** Same properties as number three. Donor should be screened for several factors. It is not mother-baby specific.

5. **Donated fresh mature or term breast milk.** Considerations same as numbers one, two and four, but may be lacking in necessary fats. Also, it is not mother-baby specific.

6. **Pasteurized donated breast milk.** Pasteurization kills harmful bacteria and viruses along with some of the good properties. It is therefore less nutritious than fresh. Retains 70 percent of protective IgA and 40 percent of lactoferrin.

7. **Fresh-frozen (lyophilization) breast milk.** Results similar to number six. Results in a decrease in total lymphocyte count and IgA concentration.

8. **Sterilized breast milk.** Must be heated to 100 degrees Celsius and the temperature maintained for twenty minutes. The sterilization process reduces thiamine and vitamin B12 binding, completely inactivates folate binding, and reduces biotin and vitamin C levels.

9. **Pre-term or specialty manufactured infant formula.** Formulated for pre-term infant. Contains necessary nutrients yet missing more than fifty-five breast milk components. Stable at various temperatures. Various formulations available, including allergy-free products. Contamination possible.

10. **Ordinary manufactured infant formula.** Difficult to digest, lacks anti-infective properties, less optimal growth and developmental gains, subject to error or contamination, more severe infections likely, wrong balance of nutrients, not mother-baby specific.

11. **Non-caloric liquids: tea or water.** Inappropriate "food" for infants. No nutrition or protection is provided.

You can see from this hierarchy that even if a mother cannot breastfeed her child, she has options available to her through pumping her own milk or using donor milk, which far exceed the inferior quality of manufactured infant formula. By now, you can see that formula and breast milk are not equivalent. Breast is best!

The United States has one of the lowest breastfeeding rates among developed countries and yet one of the highest infant mortality rates, according to data from the U.S. Centers for Disease Control. When you examine all the benefits of breastfeeding, it is clear to see how mother's milk gives babies an edge in many areas, including resistance to disease. In this chapter, we've tried to capture the "breastfeeding edge" for babies. We like to let the evidence speak for itself.

But facts alone will not bolster your resolve when self-doubt or a fussy infant threaten to derail your breastfeeding experience as you get going. There is much to learn in order to get off to a good start. It is to this process that we now turn our attention.

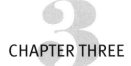

CHAPTER THREE

Getting Off to a Good Start

Getting off to a good start is a key predictor for how successfully you learn and perfect the art of breastfeeding. Your knowledge of breastfeeding, your attitude and resolve, support from others, and your perception of how things are going affect both your initial decision to breastfeed and your willingness to continue. As you gain confidence in each area, these factors should begin to work in unison. When this happens, you will be well on your way to mastering the art of breastfeeding. If these "big picture" factors collide, however, your good start and potential breastfeeding success may be jeopardized. It is worth your effort, therefore, to educate yourself about breastfeeding, gauge your own attitude and resolve toward breastfeeding in relation to the attitudes of those around you, and communicate your feelings to those whose opinions affect you.

Knowledge of breastfeeding

It is important to understand why the World Health Organization guidelines and The 2010 U.S. Healthy People Goals have been put in place. As stated earlier, these guidelines recommend exclusive breastfeeding for the first six months of life and continued breastfeeding for at least twelve months (twenty-four months in the case of the WHO) or until baby weans. Adopting these guidelines as your own is very helpful, especially as you face breastfeeding detractors. Be confident in the knowledge that a body of science has proven overwhelmingly that breastfeeding offers indisputable health, psychological, immunologic, developmental, economic, nutritional, social, and environmental advantages for babies, mothers, families, and society.

Research reveals between 50 percent and 90 percent of women decide how they will feed their babies before becoming pregnant or very early in their pregnancy. Thus, an important early step toward getting off to a good start occurs simply by making a decision to breastfeed.

Furthermore, gaining knowledge of what is normal or ought to be expected will help you recognize potential problems and seek appropriate support. This is critical because even the smallest difficulty can lead you down the path to self-doubt, causing you to abandon your resolve.

If you seek knowledge on breastfeeding from the internet, use caution. Commercial sites, government-sponsored sites and non-profit organizations all publish breastfeeding information online but it will be up to you to discern if the organization supporting a web site you are visiting is offering information in your best interests — or in theirs.

If you find yourself unsure about whether you want to breastfeed, keep learning about breastfeeding. Many women try breastfeeding without knowledge of its benefits, yet find joy in the process. While this may be fine during the first week, a woman who educates herself can muster the resolve to continue after facing one or more of the common obstacles. It's been said that attitude is everything, but attitude needs to be backed up by information, support, and experience.

Your attitude and resolve

Without realizing it, your attitude about breastfeeding is shaped in part by your race, the attitude of your peers, your level of education, your income, and according to the region of the country in which you live. After you determine your intention and begin to seek support for your decision, it will be important to understand how peoples' attitudes about breastfeeding vary; this will help you build a network that supports your decision to breastfeed, support which in turn helps build your resolve.

In the early stage of breastfeeding, it is important to set a goal for how long you plan to breastfeed, keeping in mind baby's best interests as you do. This goal will help you endure the early discomforts and inconveniences that go with breastfeeding, things you may not have anticipated. What often happens with these early goals as you learn the art of breastfeeding is baby's developmental needs supersede the purpose of your initial goal and so you set a new one. This new goal is generally not based on length of time but based on the needs of your baby. Still, the early goal will get you through the first few months if you find your resolve weakening if things are not going as you'd expected.

Deciding to breastfeed only during your hospital stay does not give you or your baby sufficient time to fully experience breastfeeding. The composition and volume of breast milk changes rapidly in the days and weeks following birth. You may experience pain — sore nipples and breast tenderness — during early breastfeeding and this may lead you to wonder if you can succeed with breastfeeding. It can only get better — and it does. The key to resolving any difficulties is to seek proper medical and breastfeeding help immediately. Don't wait for weeks or months to tick by before seeking help.

Continued breastfeeding rates will be affected by having a positive experience in these early weeks and months. In other words, chances are greater you will continue to breastfeed if you get off to a good start. But attitude also plays a role. One attitude that threatens a woman's resolve and her chance at breastfeeding success is ambivalence.

If you are ambivalent about your decision whether to breastfeed, how you will breastfeed, and for how long, it is helpful to find the root of this ambivalence. Is it merely a fear of the unknown? Are there social factors or detractors who chip away at your confidence? Do you enjoy full support from your husband, your mother, or your doctor? Do you have misconceptions about breastfeeding? Do you think breastfeeding is too much work? Are you embarrassed at the idea of breastfeeding in public? Do you perceive breastfeeding makes a social statement? Have you had a negative breastfeeding experience? Do you lack helpful resources? Must you experience breastfeeding first-hand before you can decide? Do you understand the evidence related to breastfeeding's benefits? Do you believe you should be feeding your baby only what is the best?

See the Ambivalence Checklist on pages 38-39 for ways to address some of your uncertainties. Answering some of these questions can help

AMBIVALENCE CHECKLIST
UNDERSTANDING MY AMBIVALENCE TOWARD BREASTFEEDING

Assess prior to delivery, at one week, one month, six months, and one year

Score your perceptions on a scale from 1 to 5, with 1 meaning you strongly disagree with the statement and 5 meaning you strongly agree with the statement.

SCORE	1	2	3	4	5
	I strongly disagree	I disagree	I am uncertain	I agree	I strongly agree

If you score a 3 on any statement, you appear ambivalent. If you score a 4 or 5 on any statement, taking the recommended action will help you resolve a conflict that could shore up your determination to master the art of breastfeeding. If you score lower than a 3 on any statement, you appear positioned for success.

QUESTION   **SCORE**

A.   I am *afraid* to breastfeed   _____
If you mark 4 or 5, list your reasons and seek counsel from a health care provider or certified lactation specialist.

B.   I *lack* social support from:

My husband   _____
Attend breastfeeding classes together and share this book.

My friends   _____
Discuss with friends and share this book.

My health care provider   _____
Share your concerns. Find a new provider if necessary.

Baby's maternal grandmother   _____
Share the latest facts and information.

Other family members   _____
Share the latest facts and information.

Talking about your desire to breastfeed in a non-confrontational, informational manner can help clear up misconceptions. Ask loved ones to fully support your desire to breastfeed.

C.   I don't know how to breastfeed   _____
Contact La Leche League or other competent lactation
specialists. See the appendix for contact information.
Attend breastfeeding classes.
Talk to mothers who have successfully breastfed.

D.   I had difficulty with breastfeeding   _____
Contact competent lactation specialist with a list of difficulties.*

*Determine whether difficulty was behavioral or mechanical (see page 56). If mechanical, talk to a lactation specialist to determine how to change the dynamic with this breastfeeding experience. If the problem was behavioral, breast milk comes in faster with subsequent pregnancies and may ease the fear of insufficient milk. Experience is a factor in getting off to a good start. Previous breastfeeding experience, if successful, will be helpful.

E. I need to work _____

   Assess whether this is a need or a desire.
   List priorities of your family and decisions you have made for family.

F. Breastfeeding is not for me _____

   List reasons: 1. _____

   2. _____

   3. _____

G. I don't plan to breastfeed beyond 3 months _____

   List reasons: 1. _____

   2. _____

   3. _____

H. I don't plan to breastfeed beyond 6 months _____

   List reasons: 1. _____

   2. _____

   3. _____

I. I don't plan to breastfeed beyond 12 months _____

   List reasons: 1. _____

   2. _____

   3. _____

Evaluate your reasons for questions F through I and compare them to your original breastfeeding goals. Set a new breastfeeding goal based on your current intention and the developmental needs of the baby.

If you score 3 or higher, perhaps you need to experience breastfeeding before coming to conclusions about how successful you might become. If, after reevaluating some of your concerns, you continue to score highly, keep researching or seeking professional advice. Keep in mind that strong ambivalence or opinions which detract from breastfeeding can lead others to make decisions for you and your family which you should be making.

you move past ambivalence toward determination.

Another thing to consider about ambivalence is how it might be fed by your own attitude toward family and parenthood, especially if you are expecting your first baby. How do you envision this new "family" and what role do you expect to play as parent?

You have no doubt heard about the importance of family; it is a favorite topic among politicians and the media. When researchers ask people to identify what is most important to them, nearly everyone puts family at or near the top of the list. Many people also report dissatisfaction with the quantity and the quality of time they spend with family. So the question becomes: how can people more effectively prioritize their families?

One of the things new parents can do is invest their time and energy into supporting breastfeeding. What other activity delivers families such quantifiable benefits?

Breastfeeding enables mothers and fathers to re-prioritize family needs and invest in the child who has been newly-added to the family. The role of "parent" is a true leadership role in that it allows you to influence and nurture your children using your own principles and values. Family leadership calls on you to provide for your children, protect them, nurture them, and teach them. While other family members such as grandparents, siblings, aunts, uncles, and cousins may contribute in a way, it is the leadership exercised by parents that is critical to developing a child's character. Parental leadership shapes an entire generation of new leaders; it is this ability to shape the outcome of another human being that makes parenting such an awesome responsibility and opportunity.

George Haley, former U.S. ambassador to Gambia, once said: "Much like protons, neutrons and other subatomic particles that constitute the building blocks of our physical works, the family is the cornerstone for both our social existence and individual development. It has been said it takes a village to raise a child, but I tell you it takes strong families to make a true village."

Prenatal intentions influence breastfeeding's initiation and its duration, to a point. Your initial breastfeeding experience also will influence how long you breastfeed. Behavior change is a dynamic process, especially for continuous behaviors such as breastfeeding or parenting. The information provided in this text can help bolster your early resolve, yet you will need to continue to develop your determination along the way. Certainly, if you enjoy support from others with whom you are close, it will be much easier to overcome later challenges.

Support from others

You have the greatest chance to master the art of breastfeeding when your needs and the needs of your infant are recognized and balanced. As your infant grows and develops, his nutritional and emotional needs will change. At the same time, you will face hormonal, physical, and emotional changes. Add to this the increased demands of breastfeeding within a growing family and involvement in community, and you may find your resolve weakened.

You need support from your husband, family, friends, and the community. Fortunately there are plenty of resources to which to turn for emotional and educational support. Consider how you should expect support from others in the following ways:

Emotional support comes through expressions of empathy, caring, and concern. You receive emotional support when others listen to you, agree with you or affirm your experiences; people will understand what you're going through, even if they've never experienced your exact situation. For example, your husband can offer emotional support by expressing concern for your well-being or by insuring you have adequate rest, food, and personal time. Your mother may offer emotional support by helping with the laundry or cooking. Even a simple comment such as "I recall being tired," can be Grandma's way of offering emotional support.

Esteem support comes to you through others demonstrating positive regard for your decision to breastfeed. A person who encourages you, tells you they admire your commitment, and agrees with your actions reinforces your self-esteem. Esteem support is especially critical for first-time mothers who may not have confidence in their abilities to breastfeed successfully or even to parent well. A husband who thanks and praises his wife for breastfeeding offers esteem support.

Instrumental support comes in the form of professional assistance from physicians, nurses, midwives, and lactation consultants. Instrumental support takes into account baby's measurable progress and offers ways to improve your condition or results. Instrumental support is not automatic; you will need to seek out professionals who are interested in your breastfeeding goals and want to help you achieve them.

Informational support involves you gathering as much sound advice on breastfeeding as you can, being mindful that a lot of information available on the internet or even in books may leave you confused or overwhelmed. As you educate yourself on breastfeeding, try to identify gaps between knowledge and experience, and seek out help from professionals you trust. Rely on periodicals from breastfeeding organizations such as the La Leche League to keep you up-to-date on breastfeeding information and resources.

Network support can be vital to a positive breastfeeding experience. Seek out new mothers' groups, prayer groups, or breastfeeding groups such as the La Leche League, which provide solidarity among others who share your commitment and interests. A side benefit to network support is the social outlet it offers.

Asking for assistance is something most of us need to do on occassion. Unfortunately some women are embarrassed to ask for help regarding breastfeeding or feel the knowledge should be innate. Failing to ask for help when you need it can lead to frustration, depression, and a feeling of failure. These emotions threaten your success.

Do not feel badly when you have to ask for help. Recognize when help is needed then dig deeply for the confidence required to seek the expertise you require. Even experienced mothers, when presented with new situations, will have to ask for help. Remember, excellent help is generally at your fingertips. Rely on the informational and network supports you have developed. Better yet, assemble a list of expert advisers before baby arrives, including contact information, and put the information into the Couple to Couple League's companion to this book, *The Art of Breastfeeding Diary*!

Perception of how things are going

One proven predictor of breastfeeding success is that a mother *feels* successful.

In order for you to feel successful, however, you must first understand what to expect or what constitutes *normal*, then you must see or experience normal outcomes, both in yourself and your baby. What can detract from feelings of success, even if you and your baby are experiencing normal outcomes, is holding on to unrealistic expectations. If a situation arises where you or baby are *not* experiencing a normal outcome, knowledge of what is normal puts you in a very good position to seek appropriate help. With breastfeeding, problems not quickly addressed will persist and become difficult to overcome.

The Breastfeeding Perception Assessment on page 44 is a simple way to gauge how things are going. It is a self-assessment to help you identify areas that are working well and areas you may want to improve upon. Share the results of your self-assessment with your husband, your lactation consultant, or another person in your support network for ideas on how to improve your outcomes.

Remember, a major reason for early cessation of breastfeeding is a woman's perceived difficulty with breastfeeding.

Ready, set, start: Getting ready for baby

Your choice of physician and hospital may play a role in your decision to breastfeed. When able, choose a facility and health care provider who fully supports your directives.

A recent development in maternity facilities is the Baby-Friendly Hospital Initiative, which offers an environment that fosters acceptance and practice of breastfeeding, free from the influence of infant formula manufacturers that historically have offered new mothers reduced-price coupons or products free of charge. These marketing techniques negatively impact breastfeeding rates. If you have a Baby-Friendly Hospital in your area, consider yourself fortunate; as of 2007, there were only sixty-one such facilities in the United States. (See Appendix B for a list of Baby-Friendly Hospitals.)

BREASTFEEDING PERCEPTION ASSESSMENT

Assess prior to delivery, at one week, one month, six months, and one year

Look at the outcomes below and rate them according to your perception of how well things are going. Rate each on a scale of 1 – 5, with 1 representing the lowest value and 5 representing the highest value.

POINTS	1	2	3	4	5
	Distressing	Better, but needs improvement	Satisfactory	Good	Excellent

Infant Growth

_____ Infant Growth

_____ Infant Weight Gain

_____ Baby rarely ill

_____ Baby spits up frequently

_____ Colic (adverse reactions to food mother eats)

[ ] Total points

Infant Satisfaction

_____ Infant motivated to breastfeed

_____ Infant able to breastfeed

_____ Infant response to breastfeeding/breast milk

_____ Infant seems satisfied after breastfeeding

_____ Infant enjoys breastfeeding

[ ] Total Points

Maternal Enjoyment

_____ Mother's physical comfort while breastfeeding

_____ Mothers fatigue level while breastfeeding

_____ Mother feels good about breastfeeding

_____ Mother body image while breastfeeding

_____ Mother's health is restored after birth

[ ] Total points

Maternal Role

_____ Breastfeeding provides opportunity to nurture

_____ Breastfeeding sustains infant's growth

_____ Breastfeeding increases my confidence to mother

_____ Breastfeeding helps my baby respond to me

_____ Breastfeeding helps me bond with baby

[ ] Total Points

Lifestyle compatibility

_____ Feeding schedules are easy

_____ Nighttime feedings are easy

_____ Breastfeeding limits my freedom

_____ Spouse is supportive with breastfeeding

_____ I am embarrassed to publicly breastfeed

[ ] Total points

A high value in each category shows a good balance. A low value in each indicates dissatisfaction across the board. Mixed values in various categories will point out areas of imbalance. This self-assessment should help you identify areas that are working well and areas you may want to improve upon. Share the results of your self-assessment with your husband, your lactation consultant or another person in your support network for ideas on how to improve your outcomes. Remember, a major reason for early cessation of breastfeeding is a woman's perceived difficulty with breastfeeding.

Source: Leff, E., Gagne, M. & Jefferis, S., Maternal Perceptions of Successful Breastfeeding, (*Journal of Human Lactation* 1994,) 10:2, 99–104

If you do not have access to a Baby-Friendly Hospital, there are ways to gauge whether a hospital you may be considering for delivery will support you in your resolve to breastfeed. You will want to tour potential facilities and assess the degree of support each is likely to provide. Considerations include: Does the hospital actively support breastfeeding as the preferred infant feeding method? Does it offer information or instruction on breastfeeding? Are there experienced lactation consultants or specialists available and are they certified? How actively does the staff assess and document breastfeeding for proper latch, positioning, and suck? Are these observations added to baby's medical records? Will you be allowed to initiate breastfeeding immediately after giving birth without staff interruption for non-critical procedures? Will you be encouraged to keep baby with you throughout your hospital stay, including at night? Does the hospital counsel women on breastfeeding's benefits and the risks of using manufactured infant formula? What is hospital policy regarding supplemental water or infant formula? Is there support for natural childbirth?

Additionally, your physician needs to be made aware of your decision to breastfeed and demonstrate support. If your physician is ambivalent or negative toward breastfeeding, this should be a red flag, especially when you consider both the American Medical Association and the American Academy of Pediatrics call for exclusive breastfeeding for the first six months. If your physician does not support breastfeeding, you may want to find another doctor. Talk to friends and family members for referrals to supportive health care providers in your area. Personal referrals are oftentimes the most helpful. Changing doctors may be difficult, but finding a supportive doctor is an important decision, one which you must make for the sake of your family.

A good, supportive physician can foster and influence your commitment to breastfeeding. He or she should be encouraging, supportive, helpful, and knowledgeable; he should be willing to recommend help from lactation consultants in the event you experience difficulties.

If circumstances dictate you must use a certain physician, hospital or clinic, and you find them less-than supportive, you may still control your health care. Put desires such as natural childbirth, breastfeeding, and Natural Family Planning in writing and have these directives placed in your medical file.

All set for delivery?

Medical interventions during labor and delivery often have negative cascading effects, which can hinder your progress as you begin to practice the art of breastfeeding. Medical interventions are defined as those practices and medicines designed to ease the stress of labor and delivery. Often, such practices are offered without women fully understanding how the consequence of one intervention can lead to further interventions, which may further hinder breastfeeding.

For example, one intervention used in more than 63 percent of all deliveries is the epidural drip, which is administered via a catheter into the spinal column. The first consequence from the epidural drip is a buildup of excess fluid in mother, leading to hypotension, or reduced blood pressure. For baby, the consequence of mother's epidural drip can be jaundice, feeding difficulties, and excessive water elimination postpartum, which can skew weight loss numbers, resulting in inappropriate assumptions about how well baby is breastfeeding. (Babies whose mothers received epidurals typically lost eight ounces of body weight postpartum compared to five ounces when mother did not receive an epidural).[2]

Furthermore, mother's fluid overload swells her breasts, including the area surrounding the nipple, which makes it difficult for baby to latch on properly; swelling paired with improper latch causes mother pain. In addition, epidurals have been shown to slow labor's progress, which may lead to mother receiving more medications to move labor along. A common medication given at this point is pitocin, an oxytocin derivative. The result: more swelling (edema). The effect of an epidural drip can cascade further, leading to a higher probability for delivery intervention such as the use of forceps, vacuum extraction, or even a Caesarean delivery. Vacuum extraction puts baby at risk for two life-threatening complications: head trauma and bleeding in the brain. While not every woman experiences the same negative cascading effects to this degree, the potential exists.

Narcotic interventions such as Demerol, offered to ease the pain associated with labor, likewise hinder baby's ability to effectively breastfeed after birth. Sometimes the effect lingers for days. Babies who receive narcotics indirectly from mother during labor are sleepier and less interested in breastfeeding; they can exhibit respiratory depression and inhibited sucking. Mothers also need time to recover from the effects of these drugs, further hindering mother-infant bonding and early breastfeeding. Other interventions indirectly impact breastfeeding.

Women who deliver via Cesarean birth should expect additional pain, stress and recovery time. This means initiation of breastfeeding and subsequent milk production may be slightly delayed. Finding a comfortable position in which to breastfeed will be the biggest challenge. Supportive hospital personnel will be important to breastfeeding getting off to a good start under this circumstance.

Understand that childbirth interventions are commonplace, thus they are perceived as a natural part of modern-day labor and delivery. In reality, though, these interventions are intrusive, often unnecessary, and could become an obstacle to you and baby getting off to a good breastfeeding start.

By contrast, natural childbirth eliminates drugs, and their narcotic effect, from labor and delivery. If you have taken childbirth classes and have educated yourself in natural birthing techniques, you should still expect to be offered narcotic or other pain interventions during labor and delivery. The decision whether to accept such intervention is up to you and your spouse.

Congratulations, it's a boy! Congratulations, it's a girl!

Breastfeed your new baby as soon as possible after birth; ideally feeding should occur within the first half hour, when he is incredibly alert and eager to meet you and experience his new world. Provide as much skin-to-skin contact with baby as you can manage; some suggest this contact should last for at least two hours after birth. When possible, delay unnecessary procedures until you have had a chance to breastfeed. It has been proven that early initiation of breastfeeding is associated with earlier establishment of effective sucking and feeding behaviors and enhanced mother-baby bonding. It also helps baby physiologically adapt to his new environment.

Choose a comfortable position to breastfeed. If possible, hold baby in your arms at a forty-five degree angle with baby facing your breast. A baby lying flat may have difficulty swallowing. Because of baby's size and inexperience, you will need to cup your breast and place it into his mouth. Try to get more of the lower portion of the **areola** (the darkened area surrounding the nipple) into baby's mouth. Keep your fingers off the areola; if you place all four of your fingers under the breast and your thumb on top, you will have a better chance to support the breast and help baby achieve proper latch.

Touch baby's lower lip and chin with the nipple. This action leads to an automatic reflex where baby will open his mouth wide and slightly tilt his head back. If you touch baby's upper lip, he will not respond the same way. (Test his reflex by touching both his upper and lower lip with your finger to see for yourself.) When baby opens his mouth, move him toward you, not the other way around. He should latch on perfectly.

As you repeat feedings, you will discover that it is easier to initiate breastfeeding when baby is in the drowsy, quiet alert, or active alert states. Don't wait until baby is crying; by then he is too distressed and the process is far more complicated.

It is critical to recognize when baby's latch is proper. Many women suffer sore nipples needlessly because they have not mastered the art of getting baby to latch on properly. Proper latch means baby has his mouth wide open, has flared lips and nostrils, and his cheeks and chin touch or nearly touch the breast. You should hear a sustained, rhythmic pattern of sucking, swallowing and breathing. He will pause occasionally yet he will not let go.

Initially, baby will feed for about ten minutes; allow him to feed until he is satisfied and do not stop him unless his sucking is causing you discomfort. If that's the case, remove him from the breast, burp him, and then offer the other breast. Do not worry about switching sides mid-feeding if he is eating contently and you are comfortable. Allow him to fully breastfeed on just one breast to maximize his intake of milk fat (hind milk), and then be sure to feed him on the other breast next time. After feeding, note the shape of your nipple; it should be elongated, not pinched or abraded. Correct positioning and latch will minimize nipple tenderness.

Breastfeeding your new infant will result in physiological changes with you as well. You should expect an increase in uterine contractions accompanied by a discharge of lochia, all part of the recovery process. Also, as you relax and enjoy your new child, you may find yourself overcome with emotion; you have entered a new phase of womanhood, with its inherent capacity to love and nurture another human being. Do not be surprised if your emotions leave you feeling as if you have just climbed off of a roller coaster.

Share your room with your baby twenty-four hours a day. This allows you to get familiar with his cues, which facilitates breastfeeding. Hospital staff will likely keep their distance so as not to interfere with you as you establish breastfeeding. However, if you have questions or concerns, seek out staff for help. Despite common perception, mothers whose babies share their rooms get slightly more sleep than mothers whose babies spend the night in the nursery. Furthermore, the care your baby receives in a hospital nursery may differ from the care he receives from you. Even at night, hospital nurseries are bright and noisy places.

In a twenty-four hour period, newborn babies normally breastfeed for 140 minutes. While that may seem like a lot of time, if you consider baby will likely feed at least twelve times, each feeding averages less than twelve minutes each. These are only averages, but important to be aware of during this critical time when you establish your milk supply. It is important to feed frequently and fully without regard for schedules. It is not unheard of for baby to occasionally **cluster feed**, which means he'll want two or three successive and closely-spaced breastfeeding sessions.

Cluster feeding should not be interpreted to mean mom's milk supply is unsatisfactory. Clues to whether baby is getting adequate milk supply are outlined below in Figure 3-1.

After those early days of breastfeeding, your milk will evolve from a substance called **colostrum** to more mature milk. You will know this change has occurred when you begin to experience a **let-down** reflex beginning in the first minute of feeding. Let-down is often described as a pinching or tingling sensation. Leaking breasts and engorgement, or fullness of the breasts, also occurs as breast milk matures.

Critical to getting off to a good start will be unrestricted exclusive breastfeeding because it: helps prevent breast engorgement; decreases jaundice in baby; stabilizes baby's blood sugar levels while decreasing

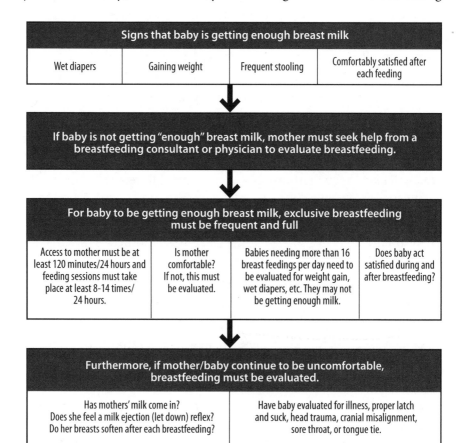

Signs that baby is getting enough breast milk			
Wet diapers	Gaining weight	Frequent stooling	Comfortably satisfied after each feeding

If baby is not getting "enough" breast milk, mother must seek help from a breastfeeding consultant or physician to evaluate breastfeeding.

For baby to be getting enough breast milk, exclusive breastfeeding must be frequent and full			
Access to mother must be at least 120 minutes/24 hours and feeding sessions must take place at least 8-14 times/ 24 hours.	Is mother comfortable? If not, this must be evaluated.	Babies needing more than 16 breast feedings per day need to be evaluated for weight gain, wet diapers, etc. They may not be getting enough milk.	Does baby act satisfied during and after breastfeeding?

Furthermore, if mother/baby continue to be uncomfortable, breastfeeding must be evaluated.	
Has mothers' milk come in? Does she feel a milk ejection (let down) reflex? Do her breasts soften after each breastfeeding?	Have baby evaluated for illness, proper latch and suck, head trauma, cranial misalignment, sore throat, or tongue tie.

FIGURE 3-1. Signs of Getting Enough Breast Milk

his initial weight loss; leads to early weight gain in baby; and allows production of mature milk to occur more quickly. It also increases your chances of achieving *long-term* breastfeeding success because milk supply is driven by demand. Dr. Paul Busam, a physician speaking on the topic of breastfeeding, put it this way: "At each feeding, the baby is not only receiving milk but simultaneously ordering his next meal."

Unrestricted breastfeeding means you will look for baby's hunger cues and address them before baby starts crying. If you attempt to restrict breastfeeding by imposing schedules or delay feedings for any reason, problems will result. Restricted breastfeeding can impede baby's ability to stool, which leads to jaundice, discomfort, and possibly more crying.

A crying baby who is not attended to quickly may use sleep as a coping strategy. In other words, babies have needs and crying is their way of saying "I needed something but you didn't notice before." Crying raises a baby's heart rate and blood pressure (by 135 percent), and impairs blood circulation in his brain. Crying also increases air intake, which causes stomach discomfort and a reduced ability to take in breast milk. Despite some common perceptions crying does not improve lung function for infants.

How will I know breastfeeding is working?

Lactation experts offer measurable outcomes for both baby and mother to help her gauge the success of breastfeeding after two weeks.[3] Positive outcomes include:

For Baby

> He is exclusively breastfeeding.

> He has regained his birth weight.

> He has at least three bowel movements in a twenty-four hour period.

> He has at least six wet diapers in a twenty-four hour period. (He'll probably exceed this number.)

> ▷ He gains approximately one ounce of body weight per day.

For Mother

> ▷ Mother is exclusively breastfeeding according to baby's feeding cues.

> ▷ She recognizes proper latch.

> ▷ Her breasts are relieved and soft after feeding.

> ▷ Breasts and nipples are pain free. Engorgement has subsided and breasts are beginning to properly self-regulate according to demand.

> ▷ Mother's perceptions match her observations. In other words, she understands the fundamentals necessary for the *art of breastfeeding* and observes success in her baby.

> ▷ Mother may experience the let-down reflex upon seeing or hearing her baby.

> ▷ Mother's fatigue has nearly peaked and will begin to recede after three to six weeks. Fight fatigue by napping when baby naps. Also, understand that fatigue is part of the postpartum recovery process for all women.

An infant who wants to feed more than sixteen times in a twenty-four hour period may not be getting enough milk. Contact a lactation consultant if this heightened demand coincides with inadequate weight gain and less-than-normal urine and stool output.

Mature milk will come in more quickly for mothers who've given birth before; for them, the process of getting off to a good start is often easier.

To supplement or not to supplement

Have you ever been counseled that babies should drink water to help flush out bilirubin, the yellow-brown pigment that normally circulates in blood and cannot be efficiently cleared by a newborn's immature liver? If so, you have been misled.

It is the caloric component in breast milk, not water, which facilitates the conversion of bilirubin to waste. Water supplements simply fill baby up while simultaneously depriving him of the calories necessary to prevent the buildup of unacceptable bilirubin levels. Frequent breastfeeding is the best way to help baby maintain lower, safer bilirubin levels. The more water a breastfed baby receives, the higher his bilirubin levels climb.

Cultural perceptions lead new mothers to believe that the longer the interval between feedings, the better. We learned in chapter two that breast milk is digested more easily and more quickly than infant formula. This means sleeping and feeding patterns among breastfed babies will not resemble sleeping and feeding patterns of formula-fed infants. It is important to understand the differences so your expectations for what is normal will match your outcomes. If you supplement in order to achieve a pattern that resembles that of a formula-fed infant, you will effectively undercut your success. When breast milk is not removed often and fully, milk production is suppressed.

Studies have shown supplementation interferes with the various stages of human milk production, disrupting maintenance of sufficient milk supply. Breastfeeding frequency and duration will quickly fall off once one or more bottles per day of formula or other supplements are introduced. The younger an infant is started on formula supplementation, the sooner he will wean from the breast. Thus, supplementation that occurs too soon will have a negative cascading effect on breastfeeding.

Supplementation is commonly introduced to prevent hypoglycemia, infant weight loss, dehydration, and hyperbilirubinemia, which leads to jaundice. Evidence supports the opposite conclusion.[4] Further evidence supports the theory that early supplementation leads to allergies, acute and chronic diseases, and other conditions later in life.[5]

Avoid the use of pacifiers, artificial nipples, or sugar-water supplements; they will impede your success. Also, do not accept free infant formula offered you at the hospital. Baby will get all the nutrition and hydration he needs from you when you exclusively breastfeed.

Frequency

You have heard it before but it is worth repeating: you will normally have sufficient milk to satisfy all your baby's requirements as long as you breastfeed according to your baby's cues. Frequent and full breastfeeding prevents sore and engorged breasts, a condition that tempts women to forestall frequent feeding, which in turn leads to decreased milk production, necessitating early supplementation, which exacerbates diminished milk supply, which eventually results in premature cessation of breastfeeding. It is a vicious cycle.

Milk production is dependent upon feeding frequency (the intervals between each session), the intensity of suck (how vigorously baby sucks), and duration of each session.

In the book *Breastfeeding: A Guide to the Medical Profession*, babies are categorized by the intensity with which they suck at the breast. The names attached to each eating "type" hint at breastfeeding behavior: Barracudas, Excited/In-effectives, Procrastinators, Gourmets, and Resters.

Barracudas latch onto the breast and suck energetically for the duration of feeding, generally ten to twenty minutes. A barracuda will put "teeth" into sucking, which may hurt his mother's breasts. Once a mother gets used to her little one's sucking action, nipple pain generally subsides.

Excited/In-effectives become so excited at the breast that they alternately grasp at the nipple, but then lose it, leading to frustration. Specialists suggest mothers try and quiet these babies before returning them to the breast. Expressing a few drops of breast milk may help excited/in-effectives focus on breastfeeding.

Procrastinators are not generally interested in feeding during the first few days; it takes a lot of sucking effort on baby's part to receive early milk. Procrastinators want to wait for the mature milk, which is easier for them to get. Maybe they are a touch lazy. Procrastinators typically do well when they are interested. Specialists recommend mothers pump after each feeding to build up milk supply, especially if procrastinators are not feeding the recommended eight to twelve times per twenty-four hour period. Even when procrastinators act disinterested, mothers should still follow hunger cues and put these babies at the breast. Furthermore, mothers should not take this disinterest personally or automatically assume there's a problem with milk supply.

Gourmets insist on mouthing or licking the nipple to taste the milk before latching. Gourmets can often be seen smacking their lips before latching. If mothers try to hurry or prod gourmets, they may become furious and fussy. Give a little gourmet the time he needs to settle down and begin to feed.

Resters will feed for a few minutes, rest a few minutes, feed a few minutes, then rest, and so on. Consequently, the duration for feeding these babies can be much longer than for others. Keep in mind, resters do not appreciate being rushed.

These descriptions serve to demonstrate how differently infants can approach breastfeeding; thus your breastfeeding management must vary accordingly. Parents need to develop a breastfeeding management plan tailored to baby's and mother's needs while also balancing the fundamentals necessary to exclusive breastfeeding, which are frequency, intensity and duration.

As baby grows and thrives, you should expect the frequency of feedings to remain high — certainly higher than the number of feedings required by a formula-fed or mixed-breastfed infant. It is important to remember all the benefits your baby is enjoying due to your commitment to exclusive breastfeeding.

Use the charts found in *The Art of Breastfeeding Diary* to track the frequency and length of each feeding. When you record actual activity, you may be pleasantly surprised to discover your perception differs from reality. Baby may be sleeping longer than you thought — especially at night — or you may not be spending as much time breastfeeding as you had perceived!

Breastfeeding management

Breastfeeding problems can be categorized into two areas, according to Linda Smith, a Board Certified Lactation Consultant. These areas are: *behavioral issues* and *mechanical issues* (see Figure 3-2, page 56).

Is milk getting into baby? *Be aware of...*

BEHAVIORAL ISSUES (80%)
...which limit access between mother and baby

Possible issues:

Illness

Inadequate time at breast

Delayed feedings

Insufficient feeding frequency

Mother-scheduled feedings

Breastfeeding attitudes

Mother's use of alcohol or tobacco

Maternal eating disorder

Watch for:

Baby unsatisfied after feeding

Mother uncomfortable

Actions:

Seek help from lactation consultant or physician

MECHANICAL ISSUES (20%)
...which limit milk flow to baby

Possible issues:

Poor latch

Improper positioning

Poor suck

Watch for:

Pain when nursing

Baby unsatisfied after feeding

Consider:

Effects of birth medication and interventions

In baby:
Tongue tie, birth trauma, cranial misalignment

In mother:
Nipple trauma, severe engorgement, post-surgery effects

Actions:

Observe, watch, and listen to baby's suck, swallow, latch, head and body positioning

Breastfeed frequently

Thoroughly dry nipples after each feeding

If not resolved:

Seek help from lactation consultant or physician

FIGURE 3-2. Is Milk Getting into Baby?

Behavioral issues include baby not having proper access to the breast for reasons that can include illness, inadequate nursing time, insufficient feeding frequency, mother's attitude about breastfeeding, mother's use of alcohol or tobacco, presence of a maternal eating disorder, or her need to schedule feedings.

Mechanical issues relate to milk not efficiently transferring from the breast to the baby. Reasons for this include: baby having problems with suck; deformity of his mouth, jaw, or tongue; hormone issues with mother including use of oral contraceptives; surgical alterations of the breast; thyroid problems, or the presence of certain cancers. In 1 percent to 2 percent of women, there exists an inability to produce a full milk supply; this is a mechanical issue.

Eighty percent of all breastfeeding problems are behavioral.[6] If baby is given the breast often enough and long enough, yet problems still exist, the problems are likely mechanical, which is helpful to know so that you seek out appropriate and specialized assistance. Early intervention is critical when addressing mechanical problems. Smith advises women who may be experiencing problems to seek out "face-to-face" intervention rather than simply relying on pamphlets or the internet.

It can be helpful if you seek out a pre-natal assessment of your breasts and nipples prior to initiating breastfeeding to avoid subsequent feeding difficulties. Most behavior issues can be resolved as long as mother is committed to breastfeeding. By contrast, not all mechanical issues can be solved.

Breast development

In most cases, mother and baby can find a happy equilibrium while maintaining exclusive or continued breastfeeding. This equilibrium can occur even after experiencing a rocky start or encountering breast difficulties, such as plugged ducts, sore nipples, tender breasts, engorgement, or mastitis. Women who experience these or other difficulties, explained in the following sections, must move quickly to identify these problems in order to resolve them and continue breastfeeding. Remember, both mother and baby must be comfortable while breastfeeding. Comfort is normal. If you find your baby is getting sufficient milk, but you are uncomfortable, you still need attention!

Before going into length about all the potential difficulties relating to the breast, let's examine how the breast works.

Breasts rarely appear as a perfectly-matched set; they often are asymmetrical and may vary in size. On average, each adult female breast weighs less than eight ounces. More significant breast abnormalities, such as breasts with unformed nipples, missing areolas or an accessory nipple, are rare and occur in less than 2 percent of the female population.

Breasts begin developing while a female is developing in the womb. Beginning at four weeks gestation, the smooth muscle of the nipple, areola, mammary buds and intricate internal channels are formed. Between thirty-two and forty weeks gestation, fetal mammary gland mass quadruples and the nipple and areola become pigmented. During childhood, breast development corresponds with general growth; structural changes do not occur until a girl reaches puberty.

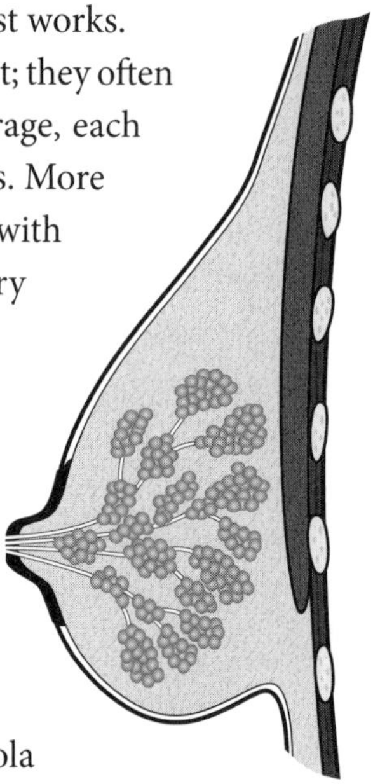

FIGURE 3-3.
Cross-section of Female Breast

At puberty, the time when ovarian function begins, structural changes to the breast also begin, thanks to an infusion of two hormones: estrogen and human growth hormone. During puberty, the primary and secondary ducts grow and divide to further develop the intricate network that includes budding and the infrastructure necessary for milk delivery.

In the accompanying Figure 3-3, notice the branching and cluster-like structure within the breast. Some say the structure resembles the cluster-like appearance of grape stems.

Beginning with puberty and continuing until approximately age thirty-five, a woman's menstrual cycle leads to further development of duct tissue in her breasts. Mammary development continues, never regressing to any former state; each menstrual cycle advances the intricate and delicate growth of the milk-delivery infrastructure of the breast. A woman's breast continues to undergo minute development with each passing menstrual cycle, even after her first pregnancy. Although these changes are minor in comparison to breast changes before and during a first pregnancy, development continues ever so slightly and intricately until a woman reaches her mid-thirties.

During pregnancy, breasts increase in size and the nipple and areola pigment darken. Lactation commences upon baby's delivery, even for pre-term deliveries that occur as early as sixteen weeks gestation. Lactation is triggered by the significant and rapid drop of progesterone that occurs once the placenta is delivered. Placental matter must be completely removed following birth; placental material is high in progesterone and even little bits left behind in the uterus can delay lactation. Key hormones such as prolactin, insulin, and hydrocortisone are necessary for lactation to commence; once lactation is underway, removal of milk is necessary for it to continue.

The gradual increase in breast size during pregnancy hints at developmental changes underway within the breast. By contrast, during lactation, the average breast doubles in weight and, again, lactation will only continue if breast milk is removed from the breast, either through breastfeeding or by pumping.

The shape of a woman's nipple can affect her perception of her ability to breastfeed. How the nipple looks when it is not in the baby's mouth does not always predict how well it will function. During suckling, the nipple elongates to double its resting length. If you are concerned about the appearance of your nipples or your potential to successfully breastfeed, seek out a lactation consultant during pregnancy for a nipple assessment. A lactation consultant can also advise you on your breastfeeding potential if you have experienced breast trauma or surgery.

Following is a discussion of some of the difficulties women who breastfeed sometimes encounter. It is important to remember that if you want to maintain milk supply, you must continue breastfeeding at the suggested frequency even while encountering any of these issues.

Leaking breasts

Leaking breasts, considered by many to be simply a nuisance issue, nevertheless present a challenge to breastfeeding mothers. Leaking occurs when the breasts are overfilled or when mother experiences a Milk Ejection Reflex (MER) brought about by external stimuli — such as the sound or sight of her baby.

Leakage due to over-filled breasts can be resolved by nursing more frequently or for longer duration. Keeping close to baby helps achieve these goals.

Mother has less control over MER and its accompanying leakage. She cannot always stop thinking about baby or may find her breasts leak when she hears another baby crying. What a mother can do is protect herself from embarrassment by preparing for leakage by wearing breast pads, which are widely available in various styles. Find one that fits your needs and always practice proper hygiene when using breast pads. If leakage occurs unexpectedly, quickly apply pressure to your breasts to limit it; you should find this technique to be effective in a pinch. (Pun intended!) Most leakage problems resolve themselves after a few months.

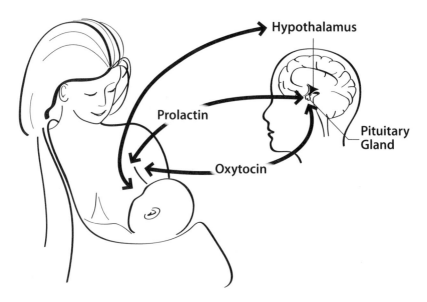

FIGURE 3-4. Milk Ejection Reflex
Source: Modified from *Breastfeeding and Human Lactation*, 3rd edition, Jan Riodan, Figure A.02.

Sore nipples

Almost all women experience some soreness or discomfort in the early weeks of breastfeeding and this discomfort is a leading cause of breastfeeding cessation. The good news is that women will adapt to the initial discomfort of breastfeeding after a few days provided baby is properly positioned and properly latched. If nipple pain persists or worsens, the most common cause is incorrect positioning of the nipple in baby's mouth.

Exacerbating nipple pain is the sometimes painful sensation accompanying let-down. As the milk flow begins each breastfeeding session, pain should subside and mother should be able to relax and enjoy breastfeeding. If pain persists throughout the feeding, however, mother should immediately seek out assistance from a lactation consultant or her healthcare provider.

The thing to remember is: *you should not feel pain while breastfeeding!* If you do, you need help.

Pinpointing nipple pain sometimes can reveal probable causes. For example, soreness on the top of the nipple, or on the tip, usually results from poor latch or improper infant tongue thrusting; sometimes the nipple is tipped too far up so that it grazes baby's hard palate. Pain on the underside of the nipple can be caused by baby stroking too vigorously on the underside of the nipple. Sometimes, mother may be supporting her breast incorrectly, which leads to improper latch. Baby should always face the breast when feeding, without being tilted or turned.

Other causes of nipple pain can be overuse of breast pumps, improper nipple care and conditioning, improper manual milk expression, pre-existing skin conditions, or a malformation of baby's mouth.

Nipple irritation left unchecked can lead to excessive dryness and the development of tissue cracking across the nipple tips. Once a nipple is damaged, simple repositioning will not be enough to eliminate pain.

Complete drying of the breast immediately after breastfeeding is important to nipple health.[7] Avoid the use of soaps, perfumes or ointments which not only dry the skin but may include scents that make it more difficult for baby to accept the breast. Wash the breasts with plain water and allow breasts to air dry. Also, change nursing pads, bras, or clothing as soon as they become wet; soaked pads can further irritate sore nipples and could also harbor bacteria. Also avoid wearing plastic backed breast pads or a bra that is too tight.

There are two types of nipple wound healing techniques recommended by lactation experts: dry wound healing, which allows for unrestricted air flow to the affected area, and wet wound healing, which works to retain moisture in the affected area. Some experts are turning to hydrogel technology in the treatment of nipple pain. Use of hydrogel pads are preferred over other topical treatments, such as lanolin, vegetable oil, petroleum jelly, vitamin E oils, antiseptics, peppermint water, and other crèmes often suggested as a remedy for cracked or damaged nipples.

Talk to your doctor or lactation consultant before using any substance on your nipple that will end up being ingested by baby. Also, seek advice from a healthcare provider should your nipple pain continue for several days, or worsen.

Breast engorgement

Breast engorgement is when breasts feel full — to the point of swelling and discomfort. Most breastfeeding mothers will likely experience some degree of breast engorgement from time to time. First-time mothers may experience engorgement more frequently and more severely. Regularly emptying the breasts through frequent and full feedings is the best prevention and management for engorgement. When milk excretion is reduced, engorgement can become an issue (milk supply too) and pain ensues.

Engorged breasts are difficult for babies to latch onto. If you experience engorged breasts, you may want to hand express milk first to soften the breast, making it easier for baby to latch. If baby does not sufficiently empty the breast, engorgement will worsen. In this case, mother might want to apply heat, gently massage or express milk to relieve pressure. A non-steroidal anti-inflammatory drug (such as Advil or Aleve) may be prescribed to improve the symptoms of engorgement.

Not all new mothers will experience breast engorgement, but many will. Here again, baby's position at the breast is important for him to maximize his feeding time. Engorgement peaks early and wanes about the second week. Once good breastfeeding habits are established, engorgement isn't likely to become an ongoing problem.

Women who've had breast implants, however, may likely suffer severe engorgement and will benefit from early lactation consultation, preferably before pregnancy occurs. If such an assessment cannot be scheduled prior to pregnancy, it should take place well before delivery and the beginning of lactation. A consultation team should include the mother's and baby's primary care physician(s), the breast implant surgeon, and a well-experienced lactation consultant. Together they should assess her chances for successful breastfeeding.

A consultation must answer more than the simple question of whether a woman with breast implants (or similar breast surgeries) will produce milk following pregnancy; they must address and fully assess whether mixed or exclusive breastfeeding is even possible. This discussion will address the current state of her breasts and implants, the types of implants used, what breast nerves were affected and remain impaired, the presence of post-surgery scar tissue, ductile blockage, and more. If it is determined that breastfeeding is possible, the medical team should put together a post-delivery plan that includes breastfeeding tips, ways to measure breastfeeding success, and resources for help when problems arise.

Plugged ducts

In addition to engorgement, tender breasts can occur from having plugged ducts.

Ducts are the passageways through which milk flows to the nipple and out of the breast; there are between fifteen and twenty-five ducts in each breast. If one or more of these ducts becomes plugged, the result will be pain, tenderness and lumpiness. Behind the point of blockage, there will be increased pressure upstream as the flow of milk slows or stops; this may lead to infection.

Breastfeeding, despite soreness, is the best treatment as the milk behind a plugged duct needs a route to the nipple. The affected breast should be completely emptied by breastfeeding or by manual expression to ease the blockage. Also apply heat before feeding or perform gentle massage to alleviate pain.

Look to an ill-fitting bra or improper feeding position as possible causes for plugged ducts. If plugged ducts become a recurring problem, seek evaluation by a lactation specialist.

Breast rashes

Rashes or sores found on the nipple or areola are unusual and often difficult to diagnose. One cause may be eczema, which is a type of dermatitis. Other causes suggest immediate medical attention.

Vasospasm

Women's breasts are very vascular, leading some women with circulation problems to experience nipple spasms. During a spasm, nipples may change appearance by blanching, or turning white, followed by a color change to blue or red before returning to normal. This cluster of symptoms is referred to as Raynaud's phenomenon of the nipple. Blanching of the nipples can occur during feeding or between feedings. Exposure to cold precipitates painful vasospasms. Relief is achieved by warming the breast. Ibuprofen, warm showers or heating pads may help alleviate discomfort.

Candidiasis

Yeast infections need attention even when side effects are mild or seem to be merely a nuisance. A yeast infection can get out of control without proper attention to become a full blown, painful infection that becomes much more difficult to treat and eradicate. While many yeast organisms can cause infection, one common culprit is called *Candida albicans*.

When yeast is present on mother's nipple, a breastfeeding baby can develop thrush. In fact, mothers with painful nipples often have infants with oral thrush. Also, a baby can get thrush after being exposed to *candida* during the birthing process, a result of yeast being present in the birth canal. If a breastfeeding baby has thrush, his mother *will* have yeast on her nipples, but not necessarily a yeast infection. Both mother and baby need to be treated simultaneously if either one hosts a yeast infection, otherwise they can pass it back and forth.

In fact, some health professionals recommend that all possible areas of infection be treated in both mother and baby. For instance, if baby has oral thrush, his diaper area needs treatment as well. If mother has a yeast infection on her nipples or breast, her vaginal area should be treated against the infection.[8] Furthermore, since yeast infection can be passed through sexual intercourse, if mother has a yeast infection in her vagina, her husband should be treated as well. Normally, babies with thrush are treated with oral medications while mothers are treated topically.

If a *candida*-like yeast organism infects mother's breasts, she can develop a painful infection that causes a burning sensation both on the skin and deep within the breast. A severe yeast infection can involve the lower ducts and sinuses of the breast in addition to skin areas. The more severe the infection, the longer it can take for treatment to work and pain to disappear. Yeast infection treatments are available either over the counter or through prescription medications. In some instances, yeast infections may call for antifungal treatments.[9] Women should consult with their physician before self-treating.

Yeast infections are often mistaken for bacterial infections or even vasospasm. Always contact a healthcare professional or lactation consultant for help with a diagnosis. In addition to advice from a competent breastfeeding professional or after consulting with a physician, consider these home remedies to help alleviate discomfort:[10]

> ▷ Expose nipples to sunlight for a few minutes each day and maximize air circulation around the breasts.

> ▷ Throw away disposable breast pads as soon as they become wet.

> ▷ Change breast pads after each feeding.

> ▷ Wear 100 percent cotton undergarments and wash them in hot water using bleach to kill *candida* spores.

> ▷ Avoid bathing with other members of the family.

▷ Restrict alcohol, cheese, bread, wheat products, sugar and honey.

▷ Ingest acidophilus daily.

▷ Rinse breasts with a lukewarm water/vinegar solution. (One tablespoon of vinegar added to one cup of water.) Breasts should be thoroughly air-dried afterward.

▷ Use ibuprofen for pain, as necessary.

▷ If advised to temporarily discontinue breastfeeding, pump frequently to maintain milk supply.

Mastitis

Mastitis is an inflammatory problem, characterized by a tender, hot, swollen, wedge-shaped area of the breast accompanied by a fever of at least 101 degrees F, chills, fatigue, and flu-like aching. Immunological factors in human breast milk protect against microbial infections for both the mammary gland and the infant, making it less likely that mastitis involves a bacterial infection. Symptoms generally last two to five days and untreated cases heal almost as quickly as treated ones. Treatments include continued and/or increased feedings at the breast, application of moist heat on the tender breast, increasing intake of fluids, rest, and/or the use of pain medication or antibiotics, if prescribed.

Lactation mastitis can occur at any time during breastfeeding and the risk of mastitis is highest among women who have breastfed previously or who have a history of mastitis. All the previously mentioned breast difficulties are risk factors for developing mastitis. Additional risk factors include:

▷ Mother experiencing stress and fatigue above and beyond normal levels.

▷ Previous breast trauma.

▷ Mother sleeping in a position that restricts circulation to her breasts.

> Maternal malnutrition or anemia.

> Illness in mother or baby.

> Rapid weaning.

After mastitis is resolved, the affected breast will produce less milk for several weeks than it did before the infection. This is normal. Do not worry that the baby will not continue to thrive. He will. Full milk production will be reestablished after healing takes place.

When a lactating woman has recurrent mastitis that does not respond to antibiotic therapy, other medical conditions may exist and intervention should be sought.

Stress and fatigue can contribute to breast tenderness and pain. New mothers can be reassured that taking daily naps with their infants is beneficial to healing and overall well-being. Proper rest promotes physical healing and gives mothers a psychological boost as well. Mothers should never equate napping with laziness. In our fast-paced world, this is often difficult advice to accept. Forget about those tales of women who waltzed out of delivery as if nothing happened. Those women are mythical.

Signs of early trouble

Breastfeeding success, even after adopting sound breastfeeding management practices, is not guaranteed. If you notice any of the symptoms listed below during the first few days and weeks postpartum, follow the accompanying recommendations:

Frequency issues

> In a twenty-four hour period, baby breastfeeds fewer than eight times or more than sixteen times. If this feeding pattern, which is outside the parameters of normal, becomes consistent and it is coupled with inadequate infant weight gain, breastfeeding may not be working properly. *Seek advice from a certified lactation consultant or a physician.*

> Mother relies on pacifiers to postpone feeding. Pacifiers and schedules adversely affect feeding frequency. Breastfeeding will suffer. *Limit or eliminate pacifier use.*

> ▷ Duration of feedings consistently is less than five minutes or longer than thirty minutes. This pattern is also outside of normal parameters; the latter may mean baby isn't getting satisfied due to insufficient milk fat or other reasons. *Seek advice from a certified lactation consultant or a physician.*

Prolonged sleeping and excessive tiredness of baby

> ▷ Baby sleeps between four and six hours a night. This can be an indication of a problem primarily in the early weeks postpartum especially if it is accompanied by inadequate weight gain, lack of wet diapers, and reduced amounts of stool. *Seek advice from a certified lactation consultant or a physician.*

> ▷ Baby consistently tires while feeding, falls asleep at the breast, and stays asleep. *If you notice this is ongoing, seek medical attention.*

Abnormal suck/swallow

> ▷ Baby's sucking is rapid with little or no swallowing. This probably coincides with baby's weight loss. *Mother needs to seek help immediately.*

> ▷ Baby pulls away from the breast, screams or cannot stay at the breast. Baby may be in pain. *Seek medical attention.*

Nipple problems

> ▷ Nipples are creased, cracked, flattened or painful after feedings. This is a sign of improper latch, which threatens continued breastfeeding. *Seek help from a lactation consultant or your health support network.*

Breast problems

> ▷ Breast fullness does not change as a result of feeding. There is likely a mechanical reason for this; *seek intervention.*

In conclusion, please consider some of the following scenarios that a breastfeeding mother might experience, along with suggestions on how to resolve the situation.

Scenario 1: Limited access

Mother and baby do not have sufficient access to one another. In other words, breastfeeding occurs for less than eight to twelve sessions (120- 140 minutes) per 24 hour period. You have learned breastfeeding frequency is critical to establishing milk supply; if access is a problem, look at possible reasons. Is mother's access limited due to baby's health issues? A lactation consultant may be able to help mother increase her access or find alternatives to exclusive breastfeeding per the feeding hierarchy listed at the end of chapter two. Baby must be adequately nourished and hydrated; limited access to mother puts baby's health at risk and prevents mother from establishing a sufficient milk supply.

Scenario 2: Uncomfortable mother

Mother and baby have sufficient access and breast milk is getting into baby but mother is uncomfortable. Mother needs to ask for advice from a lactation consultant or health care provider to help resolve her discomfort. If the discomfort is due to nipple pain, yet baby is getting adequate breast milk, mother will need advanced clinical support to as-sess and remedy the nipple trauma.

A similar scenario could play out with maternal discomfort attributed to something other than nipple pain. Again, an assessment by a lactation consultant in cooperation with a health care provider needs to occur to quickly resolve the situation. It could be mother has an infection or the discomfort is psychological. Success depends upon mother being comfortable breastfeeding.

Scenario 3: Baby isn't getting milk

Mother and baby have sufficient access to each other, but breast milk is not getting into baby. Clues include: his diaper wetting and stooling patterns, fussiness, and lack of weight gain. In this scenario, it is important to look at baby's positioning and his latch. Consult expert advice if you are uncertain whether baby is achieving proper latch.

Researchers have made great strides in their study of how an infant uses his tongue in suckling and where the infant's optimal placement is on the breast. An asymmetrical latch, where baby's mouth covers the lower part of the areola, is deemed optimal. Proper support of the breast is important.

There may be other issues affecting baby's suck, such as the residual effects of birth medications, sore throat due to aspiration, tongue tie, birth trauma, cranial misalignment*, congenital defects, or other medical problems. Again, enlist a lactation consultant or health care provider who can assess the situation and help you craft a solution.

Getting the right advice makes a difference. In 1997, for instance, one hospital classified 17 percent of its babies as reluctant feeders and reported 37 percent of its mothers complained of sore nipples. Two years later, when the same hospital achieved its Baby-Friendly Hospital accreditation, the number of reluctant feeders dropped to slightly more than 8 percent and the percent of mothers reporting sore nipples dropped to less than 11 percent. By the time this same hospital was reaccredited in 2004, both figures had fallen below 3 percent. During the same time period, the proportion of mothers who abandoned breastfeeding in the first ten days postpartum fell from 25 percent to 5 percent.

You can see, therefore, how important it is to get good breastfeeding advice, and seek help early when experiencing difficulty, or even mere uncertainty. If you have built your support network and are willing to use it, you and baby should be off to a good start, and well on your way to mastering the art of breastfeeding!

---

* Cranial misalignment is caused by normal birthing processes or by instrument deliveries using such devices as forceps, suction and vacuum extractors. At birth it is common for baby's major cranial bones to override each other; this happens as baby's head is compressed while pushing through the cervix and vagina of mother's body. After birth, these bones normally realign properly. If they don't realign properly and continue to "over-ride" each other, baby can become fussy, cry frequently and is less able to be comforted and soothed. His suck may be affected as well as he reacts to head pain and discomfort while sucking. One study found that osteopathic treatment offered symptom relief after birth.[14] Parents concerned about this should consult with a Doctor of Osteopath or their baby's physician.

CHAPTER FOUR

Bonding, Proximity and Bed-sharing: The Issues

In the last chapter, you learned how important it is to stay in close proximity to baby as you begin to learn and practice the art of breastfeeding. If at all possible, baby should begin suckling at the breast within minutes of birth and you and baby should share a hospital room throughout your stay. Twenty-four hour access to baby helps you learn his hunger and nurturing cues; close proximity facilitates your immediate response to those cues, which serves to reassure him. Being close to you also helps him reconnect with your rhythmic environment, which he enjoyed during his fetal experience. It is this close and immediate interaction between mother and baby, allowed through breastfeeding and sharing room space, which facilitates bonding, jump-starts milk production, and gets you off to that all-important good beginning.

New mothers are encouraged to take advantage of hospital time, with its lack of outside distractions, to bond with baby. (Mothers who give birth at home are encouraged to limit early distractions for the same reason.) Upon hospital discharge, it is important to not let household responsibilities threaten your newly-formed connection to baby or how well you interpret his cues. In other words, do not allow your return home to impede breastfeeding success. Even at home, you must continue responding to him promptly. Frequent, exclusive and unrestricted breastfeeding is necessary to build and maintain milk supply; it also fulfills baby's need to feel secure and loved in his new environment.

One challenge many breastfeeding mothers must overcome is fatigue, which can be exacerbated by lack of sleep and a return to household responsibilities. When you commit to breastfeeding you are consigning yourself to become the sole source of nutrition for your infant, and for good reasons.

This does not preclude your husband's direct help with day and night feedings, however, and it does not mean that men are "off the hook." A loving husband and father will come to realize that he can assist his wife in other ways. Be willing to accept his help, even if his way of doing things differs from yours. If your husband appears to be overwhelmed, he probably is! Women are not the only ones facing challenges after birth and throughout breastfeeding; husbands and wives must continue to work on their communication, help each other cope with daily challenges and move forward together.

If your husband is at a loss for ways to help out, suggest that he bring the baby to you for feedings, change the baby's diapers before and after feeding, help you get comfortable, do laundry or the dishes or help out with any older children.

In the early weeks, baby will feed frequently twenty-four hours a day, meaning you will face an interrupted sleeping pattern. Soon, you may wonder if breastfeeding will ever allow you a full night's sleep. The answer is yes, but there are steps necessary for you to take in order for this to occur; furthermore, there are developmental stages baby must pass through before he develops a more mature sleep pattern that mirrors yours. The art of breastfeeding allows you to instill in baby such a pattern, allowing for longer periods of night rest for you both. To this end, close proximity to baby, day and night, remains critical as you transition from hospital to home.

During baby's fetal development, he is connected to your biorhythms, which include temperature maintenance and wake-sleep patterns. At birth, this physical connection was lost and his immature system is unable to reestablish biorhythms encountered in the womb. Establishment of mature biorhythms is an essential marker of infant development. Your household likely has pre-established sleep-wake patterns affected by external forces such as light, social activity and eating, and internal forces, which are inherited or genetically predetermined. Exclusive breastfeeding enables baby to synchronize his patterns to those of the household. These practices hinge on maintaining a close proximity to baby, even during the night.[1]

Welcoming baby home

A common reaction to a first pregnancy is to put time, effort, and resources into creating a nursery space for baby. Couples will paint, decorate and furnish this space out of a baseless assumption that baby requires independence and solitude in order to thrive. Yet baby does not need a crib set up in a separate room down the hall in order to thrive; baby needs close proximity to his mother, which facilitates exclusive breastfeeding, frequent nurturing, touch, and interaction. Furthermore, mother does not need to be traipsing down a long hallway to the nursery, turning on lights, and sitting in a rocking chair to feed at two o'clock in the morning. Such activity upsets her biorhythms, making it more difficult for her to return to sleep. And, this does nothing to establish a more mature biorhythm in baby.

Normal newborns will have irregular sleep patterns during the first six months. During a twenty-four hour period, the average newborn will sleep sixteen or more hours; this sleep however, comes one or two hours at a time. As sleep patterns mature, infants will begin to sleep for longer stretches as the total number of hours they sleep decreases. It will be important for the well-being of everyone in your household for your infant to learn that longer periods of sleep should occur during the night. Keeping baby close at night helps accomplish this goal.

When mother and baby sleep in proximity to one another, their closeness allows them to achieve synchronicity in body temperature control and sleep-wake patterns. Sharing sleeping space offers other benefits.[2] Mother can hear baby breathing and rest better knowing he is within reach if a problem develops; mother and baby get better rest, which can impact their temperaments, which in turn, improves how they interact. Sharing sleeping space also provides mother and baby physiological benefits. Adequate sleep, along with good nutrition and exercise, is a key factor for maintaining good health. A healthy, well-rested mom is less likely to view exclusive breastfeeding as a disproportionate burden as she continues to be the sole provider of infant nutrition.

Sharing sleeping space can be accomplished in several ways. Some new parents will bring their baby right into bed with them for the entire night. This arrangement works best if you have a large bed. Other couples will go to sleep in their bed without baby, but will bring him into bed for his first night feeding and leave him there for the remainder of the night. Some couples use side sleepers, which attach to the side of an adult bed, allowing them to maintain closeness while giving each their own sleeping space. Some people simply place a bassinet or cradle for baby in their bedroom. All of these arrangements facilitate nighttime breastfeeding and allow baby to sync with mother sooner than if he were sleeping in a nursery elsewhere in the home. You and your husband should decide which sleeping arrangement works best for your family.

Considerations of sharing night space

For the first weeks of life, human babies are unable to efficiently regulate their body temperatures without close proximity to other humans. This is why babies left in hospital nurseries are often wrapped tightly in blankets and have hats placed on their little heads. Deprived of closeness with other humans, babies cannot thrive; human babies need to connect with other humans during the day and at night in order for them to develop the ability to regulate their own temperatures and other important biorhythms. Body temperature regulation is the earliest circadian rhythm to develop in human babies; it is the first step toward developing mature sleep-wake patterns. Furthermore, babies need to smell, touch, hear, and feel their mothers in order to direct their energy into growth or maintenance. All of these earliest developmental needs are effectively met by applying the principles behind the art of breastfeeding.

Breastfeeding allows baby to be close to mother, to hear her, to touch her, and to connect to her breathing patterns. All of these things help him advance developmentally.

How mother nurtures during the day, however, will differ from how she meets his needs during night feedings. External activities such as light, sound, and social interaction can affect how baby develops his natural body rhythms; these stimuli ought to be reserved for daytime feedings and playtime. Daytime interactions that create in baby a desire to play become problematic at night as you attempt to get his sleep pattern to match yours.

Daytime feedings and playtime offer you adequate opportunities to stimulate baby. As you practice the art of breast-feeding, expect to be overcome by the desire to touch, hold, stroke, massage, and gaze at baby. These feelings will not disappear at night. Understand, however, that feedings during the night should be done silently and without external stimuli. If baby sleeps in close proximity to you, it will be easier for you to meet his needs before he wakes fully and be-comes distressed. If you sleep in separate rooms, it will be more difficult for you to re-spond in a way that allows both of you to get back to sleep quickly.

The art of breastfeeding should allow for the natural and gradual establishment of sleep-wake rhythms so that baby will learn that night-time is sleep time and daytime is playtime. Until this is accomplished, mother is well-advised to nap during the day to catch up on sleep missed during night feedings.

Keeping baby close does not automatically mean baby shares your bed, but if he does, be aware that there are safety risks inherent in shar-ing an adult bed with a baby. The American Medical Association points to a U.S. Consumer Products Safety Commission study, which reported 515 infant deaths resulted from sharing a bed with a parent, sibling, or other adult between 1990 and 1997, as reason enough to avoid placing children under age twenty-four months in an adult bed. This particular CPSC study, however, has been challenged by a number of healthcare professionals who state it is impossible to know how many infants sleep in adult beds, for how long, and what other contributing factors such as the use of drugs or alcohol were present in the reported cases. Without knowing all the facts, the numbers lack clear meaning.[3]

The American Association of Pediatrics takes a more neutral stance with regard to baby sleeping in an adult bed. It states that there is insufficient data to conclude that such an arrangement is neither hazardous nor safe; in the view of the AAP, certain conditions make such an arrangement hazardous. These conditions include: the presence of loose covers, a bed pushed against a wall, a non-parent in bed with the baby, and parental use of drugs, including alcohol and tobacco. Bed sharing can also be problematic if one or both parents are obese or suffer from severe sleep disorders such as restlessness or sleep apnea.

James McKenna, a noted sleep expert and author of *Sleeping with your Baby*, says the notion that a baby ought to sleep isolated from his parents coincided with the twentieth century promotion of infant formula as superior to breastfeeding and the belief that minimizing nighttime touch between parents and infants resulted in the development of normal infant sleep patterns. Pediatric icon Dr. Benjamin Spock reinforced this position; he promoted independent sleeping as an ideal which resulted in adults with good sleep practices and good hygiene. Still others said allowing a baby to share a bed with his parents could lead to sibling rivalry, sexual or emotional confusion, over-stimulation, bad habits, and marital discord or divorce. No evidence of these effects has been proven through study; furthermore, numerous studies conducted since 1990 have completely refuted these beliefs. One expert who actively promoted infant isolation at night has since expressed regret over his statements.[5]

If you and your husband determine that placing baby in bed with you is the most convenient way to stay in close proximity, there are several things you can do to help insure baby remains safe, including:[6]

> ▷ Baby should sleep supine, meaning on his back.

> ▷ Avoid beds with soft surfaces such as water beds, pillow-top mattresses, and featherbeds. Pillows, stuffed animals, comforters and quilts, sheep skins, bean bags, and other soft items

sometimes found in beds have been found to contribute to the deaths of young infants.

▷ Be certain that no gaps exist between the mattress and the bed frame. Infants and even small children can become wedged in gaps and asphyxiate.

▷ Bedding should fit snuggly around the mattress. Sheets that slip from a corner can smother a baby.

▷ Parents and infants should avoid strings or ties on all night clothes; these pose a strangulation risk.

▷ Avoid the use of loose coverings where baby is sleeping.

▷ Keep baby's face uncovered to allow ventilation.

▷ Avoid smoking. Exposure to tobacco is associated with a higher risk of Sudden Infant Death Syndrome.

▷ Avoid overheating the room in which the baby sleeps and avoid overdressing baby. Overheating is associated with an increased risk of Sudden Infant Death Syndrome.

▷ Keep the bed away from window treatment cords or sashes. These pose a strangulation risk.

▷ Very long hair should be pulled back and fastened. Baby can become entangled and strangle in very long hair.

▷ Railings used in head boards or foot boards should be spaced no farther apart than those in safety approved cribs: 2-3/8 inches.

▷ Refrain from using a side rail with infants under twelve months of age. Babies can become wedged between the mattress and the side rail resulting in suffocation.

▷ Do not put baby to sleep alone in an adult bed.

▷ Avoid entrapment. Move the bed away from the wall and

other furniture and avoid placing baby in a bed that presents an entrapment hazard.

> Only parents are advised to sleep with their baby. Other adults, children, or siblings should avoid bed sharing with infants. All have been identified as increasing the risk of infant suffocation.

> Parents who smoke or have consumed sedatives, medications, alcohol, or any substance that causes altered consciousness or marked drowsiness should not sleep in the same bed as an infant.[7]

> Extremely exhausted parents should avoid bed sharing with baby until they are more rested; unresponsiveness from extreme fatigue increases suffocation risk.

> Avoid sharing a bed with baby if either spouse is ill.

> Avoid sharing a bed with baby if either spouse is markedly obese.

> Avoid placing an infant in bed with pets.

If you and your husband decide to keep baby close at night, but not place him in your bed, use only safety-approved infant sleeping products and take note of these cautions:

> Do not sleep with baby on a sofa or an overstuffed chair.

> Baby should not sleep in a car or infant seat as they fail to adequately support the infant's upper body. This can cause blockage of the baby's airway, putting him at risk for suffocation.

> Eliminate pillows and stuffed animals from baby's crib or cradle.

> Don't use padded crib bumpers or quilted comforters.

> Make sure the mattress is firm.

> Be sure to measure crib slats so that they are no more than 2-3/8 inches apart. Familiarize yourself with other safety standards of infant sleeping products.

> Keep cribs and cradles away from drapery cords or other strangulation dangers.

> Examine baby's sleeping arrangement with an eye to safety.

> Don't overdress baby.

> Always place a sleeping baby on his back.

Infant cribs must meet safety standards while adult beds are not held to such guidelines. This means parents must be extra vigilant to examine their sleeping space with an eye to safety. Not every couple will share their bed with their baby every night, yet almost every parent reports having shared their bed with their child at least once by the time their baby reaches the age of three.[8]

Studies have revealed that sleep safety issues are real. Babies have suffocated in parent beds. They have also been entrapped by headboard or walls. Thus for the best interests of the family, pay attention to these safety recommendations.

Sudden Infant Death Syndrome

Sudden Infant Death Syndrome (SIDS) is the term attached to *unexplainable* deaths of babies under the age of twelve months. SIDS was formerly referred to as crib death. The term SIDS is applied only as a cause of infant death once a thorough investigation is completed (including a complete autopsy, examination of the death scene, and a review of the infant and family clinical history) and no other cause can be determined. In 1969, scientists coined the term SIDS and recognized it as a distinct disease — little comfort to bereaved parents left with few answers as to its actual cause.

The Academy of Breastfeeding Medicine points out in its Protocol Number Six that coroners examining SIDS victims have no way to differentiate between actual SIDS deaths and accidental or intentional smothering. This is problematic as it has led many coroners to assign cause of infant death occurring in a crib to SIDS while assigning cause of death occurring in an adult bed to smothering. This leaves the impression that it is far more dangerous for baby to sleep in his parent's bed than in his own crib. This is a skewed interpretation of the facts.

It is well-regarded that several factors are linked to the occurrence of SIDS. None of these factors could lead to the conclusion that a crib is safer than sleeping with a parent. Some of the risk factors associated with SIDS are included in the book *The History of Sudden Infant Death Syndrome*, by Julia Mahler, and are offered here:

> **Time of day:** SIDS is associated with sleep and one study revealed that 50 percent of all victims die between midnight and eight o'clock in the morning, 36 percent die between eight o'clock in the morning and four o'clock in the afternoon, and 14 percent die between four o'clock in the afternoon and midnight.

> **Time of year:** SIDS is associated with sharp temperature drops and the winter season.

> **Time of life:** Most SIDS victims are between three weeks and twelve months in age. SIDS peaks at two months to three months and is extremely rare after five months.

> **Gender:** SIDS victims are 60 percent male, 40 percent female.

> **Tobacco use:** SIDS is associated with maternal tobacco use during and after pregnancy. Tobacco harms brain development in a developing fetus.

> **Sociology:** The SIDS rate is higher for economically disadvantaged families and for non-caucasions.

> **Birth weight:** Low birth-weight infants are more susceptible to SIDS.

> **Birth order:** First-born infants are less likely to die from SIDS as later-born babies.

▷ **Bedding:** Soft pillows are found to have a much higher association with SIDS than hard, flat ones. Large bed quilts also have been known to suffocate babies.

▷ **Sleeping position:** Infants placed on their stomachs to sleep are at higher risk for SIDS than infants sleeping on their backs. Furthermore, infants accustomed to sleeping on their backs, but placed on their stomachs, have a greater risk for SIDS.

▷ **Food-borne illness:** Botulism has been discovered in 5 percent or more of SIDS cases. Honey, oftentimes used on pacifiers or rubber nipples, is a proven source of botulism.

▷ **Temperature:** Evidence points to excessive heat involved in SIDS cases. Many victims have been discovered excessively dressed or covered.

▷ **Feeding:** Exclusively breastfed infants have less incidence of SIDS than never breastfed infants.

Studies have shown that breastfeeding offers a protective edge against the risk of SIDS. *The International Journal of Epidemiology*, published in 1993, found a "reduced risk for SIDS in breastfeeding infants and this reduced risk persisted during the first six months" after researchers accounted for variables such as maternal, demographic, and infant factors. The incidence of SIDS drops dramatically after age six months. Furthermore, exclusively breastfed infants have a significantly reduced risk of SIDS over infants who are mixed feeders or those who never breastfed.

In addition to breastfeeding providing a protective edge against SIDS, infant sleeping position has been shown to be important. The Back to Sleep program, launched jointly in 1992 by the AAP and the AMA, recommends placing infants on their backs (supine) while sleeping to reduce the risk of SIDS. Since this promotional effort was launched, the number of infants sleeping face down has decreased to 20 percent from 70 percent *and* SIDS has dropped by 40 percent.[9] Research also indicates the Back to Sleep program allowed for a proportional decrease in the association between SIDS and the winter season. The Back to Sleep program has since been extended worldwide. In many Asian cultures where breastfeeding and sleeping in close proximity to baby are the norm, incidences of SIDS are rare.

The exact cause of SIDS remains elusive and opinions on its roots have changed over time as the list of risk factors grows long. Research is ongoing. Some researchers note that SIDS victims have delayed development of the brain stem which controls heart rate, deepness of sleep, and breathing patterns.[10] This hypothesis supports the need for infants to remain in close proximity to mothers, especially at night, as they age and entrain their biorhythms while also supporting the need for proper nutrition necessary for brain development. Again, there is no better way to accomplish these goals than through the practices you are developing through the art of breastfeeding.

Attachment parenting, ecological breastfeeding and co-sleeping

Exclusive breastfeeding means that up until age six months, baby gets 100 percent of his nutrition from breast milk. It is characterized by frequent and full breastfeeding, offered day and night according to baby's cues; this breastfeeding pattern offers the best opportunity to achieve breastfeeding success because it allows for maximum milk synthesis based on supply and demand. No supplements of any kind, solid or liquid, are offered. Mother breastfeeds according to baby's cues for hunger and nurturing.

Mixed breastfeeding means a mother will provide, along with breast milk, supplemental foods or liquids before six months of age. Mothers who provide 100 percent of infant nutrition through pumped breast milk are also considered mixed breast feeders because suckling provides more nipple stimulation than pumping, leading to increased milk synthesis.

Babies will normally require additional caloric intake beginning at six months. Foods that provide the additional calories over and above what breastfeeding provides are termed **complementary foods**. Complementary foods do not replace breastfeeding frequency or intensity or breast milk calories. The term "complementary foods" is not synonymous with the term supplementary foods.

Supplementary foods replace some of the calories previously provided through breastfeeding, leading to a decline in breastfeeding intensity and frequency, and eventual weaning. Breastfeeding can be enjoyed by mother and child for many months (perhaps even a year or more) beyond when mother introduces supplementary foods into her baby's daily feeding regimen. Weaning does not have to closely follow the introduction of supplementary foods.

Continued breastfeeding is the term applied to mothers who continue to breastfeed after their baby reaches age six months, regardless of whether they also employ complementary or supplementary feedings.

All of these terms were defined by experts in the field of lactation and their use is important because universal nomenclature is critical to any discussion and analysis of breastfeeding. The term "breastfeeding" by itself isn't sufficient to describe the various types of breastfeeding behavior. These terms also will become important as we learn how breastfeeding impacts the return of postpartum fertility.

Other terms sometimes used in the realm of breastfeeding discussion include: ecological breastfeeding, attachment parenting and co-sleeping.

Ecological breastfeeding was promoted by The Couple to Couple League since its early years. Ecological breastfeeding was defined by seven standards: exclusive breastfeeding; pacifying baby at the breast (no bottles or pacifiers); sleeping with baby for night feedings; sleeping with the baby for a daily nap feeding; breastfeed frequently day and night; avoid schedules, and avoid any activity that restricts breastfeeding or separates mother from baby. The basic principles of ecological breastfeeding are frequent and unrestricted breastfeeding (day and night), a primary factor in producing natural lactational amenorrhea (infertility).

The Couple to Couple League continues to encourage the principles behind ecological breastfeeding because they are best for baby and mother. For instance, frequent and exclusive breastfeeding during the first six months not only helps establish and maintain adequate milk supply, it provides the big eight health benefits discussed earlier. Pacifiers, schedules, and limited contact with baby reduce the frequency of breastfeeding and interfere with the establishment and maintenance of adequate milk supply. The Couple to Couple League no longer uses the term ecological

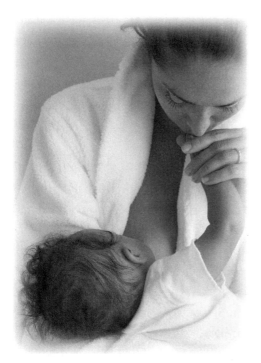

breastfeeding, however, because the term is not widely accepted nor understood among breastfeeding experts.

Furthermore, research on lactational amenorrhea has revealed factors which affect a woman's fertility beyond those associated with ecological breastfeeding. Women who practice the seven standards of ecological breastfeeding can experience an early return to fertility; when this happens, they can feel like they have not breastfed correctly or are not as good at breastfeeding as women who experience lengthy amenorrhea. (You will learn more about lactational amenorrhea and how it affects the return of fertility in chapter seven.)

Attachment parenting is a term with multiple connotations which may or may not link to breastfeeding. Attachment Parenting International offers eight principles as the foundation for attachment parenting. They are: preparing for pregnancy, birth and parenting; feeding with love and respect; respond with sensitivity; use nurturing touch; engage in nighttime parenting; provide consistent and loving care; practice positive discipline; and strive for balance in personal and family life.

The Attachment Parenting International web site includes the following statement on infant feeding: "newborn's rooting, sucking and crying reflexes evolved to ensure the close proximity of a mother or other caregiver that the baby can depend on to meet her intense needs." Also on the Attachment Parenting International web site is a list of appropriate bottle nursing practices; including this statement: "feeding is one of the primary ways a mother can initiate a secure attachment relationship with her baby. Familiarize yourself with breastfeeding behaviors and model them when bottle feeding." While the principles promoted by Attachment Parenting International are laudable, their principles are not synonymous with the art of breastfeeding.

Co-sleeping is a term often used in conjunction with exclusive breastfeeding; its connotation is that mother and baby share one bed. However, there are organizations and products that use the term co-sleeping to mean mother and baby simply sleep in close proximity, not in the same bed. Because the term is used to mean different things by various groups, it is problematic to apply the term co-sleeping to a discussion on the art of breastfeeding.

While many people can become attached to terms or rely on them to convey a certain message, it is important that terminology be universally accepted in medical and academic circles without ambiguity. When terms have varied meanings depending upon perspective or affiliation with a certain group, knowledge, communication, and understanding ultimately suffers.

Each baby brings his own needs to the breastfeeding relationship and each couple should respond to those needs in a way that best suits their family's goals and values. The art of breastfeeding cannot, nor should it, prescribe parenting practices.

Furthermore, while select breastfeeding activity has the ability to extend postpartum infertility, it is not the role of this book to advise women to breastfeed for the sole purpose of spacing babies. (An in-depth discussion of lactational amenorrhea can be found in chapter seven). Therefore, while it is important to establish breastfeeding frequency and intensity at a level that meets baby's requirements, how you attach to baby, day and night, is best left for parents to decide for themselves.

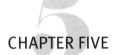

CHAPTER FIVE

Breastfeeding "Buttinskies"

As a young mother with a growing family, I often encountered people who looked upon our large family negatively. Sometimes, their comments stung and left me discouraged. When I shared with my neighbor, an elderly Czech immigrant, distress over these uninvited comments he would always smile and wave his hand as if brushing aside a gnat. "Don't let those 'buttinskies' get to you," he advised. "God knows what's best for your family."

Buttinsky is Czech slang for a troublesome meddler or one who officiously interferes with the actions of others. When you encounter someone who offers you an unwelcome opinion on your decision to breastfeed your child — you've encountered a *breastfeeding buttinsky*.

You can classify as a buttinsky any of the following: a passerby who tosses you a stern stare as you discreetly breastfeed in public; a societal standard that promotes baby's independence sooner than he's ready; a corporate policy that makes it difficult for you to continue breastfeeding after you've returned to work. Any opinion, comment or policy that negatively impacts your resolve to exclusively breastfeed (neither solicited nor welcomed) could be considered a breastfeeding buttinsky.

You've learned that breastfeeding is successful when mothers' and infants' needs are recognized and balanced. The process of recognizing and balancing needs is dynamic. One must factor together baby's physical and neurological development and his nutritional and his emotional needs, then also consider mother: her changing body, her periodic hormone shifts, her emotions, and the increasing demands placed on her by family and the community. Success comes through recognizing the process of change underway in both mother and baby and adapting circumstances to promote a mutually satisfying breastfeeding experience. Despite growth, change and adaptation, if mother evaluates the breastfeeding experience positively from birth to baby-led weaning, we can consider her proficient in the art of breastfeeding.

When social, political, corporate, personal, medical, and sexual attitudes align to support breastfeeding, the number of women who initiate breastfeeding increases and breastfeeding cessation rates fall. When these same external forces oppose women's efforts to give their babies the optimum food choice, breastfeeding initiation rates drop and cessation rates rise. Like it or not, the direct and implied messages about the value of breastfeeding that permeate the culture create certain paradoxes influencing women away from doing what is best for their babies.

What many women will discover as they start down the breastfeeding continuum is that they'll be showered with support in the early weeks. But in a few months, this support wanes, replaced by encouragement to hurry the little one along toward independence. It will be fine with just about everyone that you breastfeed a six-week-old, but some will tell you your six-month-old child won't be harmed if he starts drinking cow's milk from a cup and still others will be more than happy to order your twelve-month-old a Happy Meal from McDonalds! A twelve-month-old at the breast will shock more people than a twelve-month-old with a fist-full of French fries.

The social, political, corporate, personal, medical, and sexual influences that chip away at your resolve to exclusively breastfeed will increase the longer you breastfeed. As it does, and as you struggle to hold onto your resolve in the face of such detrimental influences, turn to your greatest breastfeeding ally, the one who shares your home — your husband.

In studies of breastfeeding mothers, the results of which are published in the *Journal of Human Lactation*, when asked to identify who provides the most support for their decision to breastfeed, mothers most often point to their baby's father. Conversely, when fathers are unsupportive of breastfeeding, women are more apt to feed their babies manufactured infant formula.

Paternal support

Paternal support is critical to achieving breastfeeding success. Your baby's father should be encouraged to learn how breastfeeding benefits baby, you, and your family. In the same research conducted on paternal attitudes toward breastfeeding, some fathers reported they felt "expected to support breastfeeding without having sufficient knowledge or understanding of how breastfeeding works." If father's influence over your potential success is more powerful than your doctor's, your mother's, or your lactation consultant's, it makes sense for him to become as knowledgeable as possible on the topic of breastfeeding.

Baby's father should be made aware that his attitude about breastfeeding will affect your own, including your decision whether to initiate breastfeeding, and for how long you plan to continue. Because his role as your parenting partner is so significant, encourage him to express his feelings about breastfeeding, including how breastfeeding affects his sexual attraction toward you. Don't avoid these discussions and don't assume he's automatically supportive or unsupportive. You shouldn't have to guess at his feelings as you watch him watching you breastfeed his baby. Ask him what he's thinking and talk about any outside negative influences each of you encounter. Remind him that it is his understanding, support, and assistance that helps you both keep breastfeeding buttinskies at bay. After all, baby is depending upon both of you for his best possible outcome. You can, and should, become a breastfeeding team!

Sadly, society sometimes encourages women to push fathers aside when making important child care decisions. Excluding father from learning about breastfeeding can impact his adjustment to the process; he must be adequately prepared for

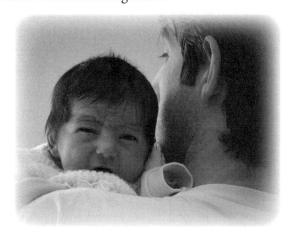

the demands of breastfeeding so that he can avoid feelings of exclusion and envy. It is important for both mother and father to understand that breastfeeding is not always sunshine and daisies. There will be stresses. If each of you approaches breastfeeding realistically, the chances of being derailed by a negative experience will be reduced.

As is common with researchers, fathers participating in a study, reported by the *Journal of Obstetrics, Gynecologic and Neonatal Nursing*, were "typed" according to their attitudes about breastfeeding. These fathering types that emerged include: Involved, Assistors, Supervisors and Detached.

Involved fathers actively participate in the decision to breastfeed and step up their efforts at home to help care for baby and other children in the home.

Assistors allow their wives to take the lead regarding breastfeeding and get involved in caring for mom, baby and other children. What differentiates an Involved from an Assistor is how each might approach breastfeeding when mother's resolve to continue weakens. An Involved will likely encourage mother to push forward for the sake of baby while an Assistor will have trouble encouraging his wife to continue breastfeeding if she encounters difficulty.

Supervisors are fathers who are involved with the decision to initiate breastfeeding but who provide little in the way of household assistance or support. Supervisors like the "idea" of breastfeeding but don't put any effort toward making it successful.

Finally, **detached** fathers do not get involved in child care or breastfeeding decisions.

Just as mothers need to adapt to the changes brought about by breastfeeding, so do fathers. It may be helpful to understand several stages men go through as they travel along the breastfeeding continuum.

First, a man must **become aware** of breastfeeding's impact on him, on his wife and on baby. Often, this awareness comes from the realization that breastfeeding isn't always the most convenient way to feed baby. Perhaps this conflicts with early assumptions, which are now being dispelled. Reality can strike a father when he realizes breastfeeding is hard work.

Secondly, a father will **adopt coping strategies** to make breastfeeding more acceptable or workable for him. For instance, he may draw on facts such as: breastfeeding cannot be duplicated, formula feeding can be dangerous to baby's health, or that *he* is now the primary beam of support for his wife. He also comes to realize that breastfeeding does not last forever.

In the next stage, a man will **discover** that his observations do in fact reinforce his knowledge. For instance, a father will observe his baby is healthy and vigorous, which he attributes to breastfeeding. Also, he may begin to enjoy the economics of breastfeeding.

The next stage is one of **compensating**, when a father increases his interaction with his infant after he realizes that bathing, changing diapers, rocking, holding, cuddling, talking to baby, putting baby to bed and comforting baby are all ways he can express fatherhood. He may even encounter situations when he can provide comfort when mother cannot. Father to the rescue!

Finally, father enters the **catching up** phase, which occurs post weaning. This is when a father finds himself the center of his child's attention, a dramatic change from when baby identified more closely with his food source — his mother. Father's importance as a parent becomes even more significant if a new infant has entered the family by this time.

Men are called by God to learn that being a father (being masculine) is different from being a mother. Men must learn and define their fatherly role; they should not merely imitate the roles assumed by their wives or mothers or wish they could be like mother. Furthermore, men must become leaders for their families. When fathers assume leadership of their families, they take on the roles of protector, defender, and yes, even nurturer. By staying open to how they must develop into the masculine role of father, men love more fully as God loves, and they come to understand that they must pass that love along to their wives and children. In this fashion, men do their part to fulfill God's will for the human family.

External forces working against you

When social, political, corporate, medical and sexual attitudes align to support you in your decision to breastfeed, you have a greater chance to appreciate and enjoy the art of breastfeeding. Chances are great, however, that you will receive mixed messages regarding the benefits and practicality of continued breastfeeding; conflicting attitudes and policies lead you to several paradoxes.

Should you ignore the prevailing attitudes of society and continue breastfeeding knowing you are doing the best thing for your baby and your family? If you do, you may find yourself incorrectly labeled "lactivist," one who engages in in-your-face activities to make the point that breastfeeding should be widely accepted. Or, do you cave into external forces in order to conform, thereby depriving yourself and baby of critical health, developmental, nutritional, environmental, immunological, psychological, economic and social benefits?

Moreover, will you accept God's design for your female body, which allows you to nurture and sustain another human person?

If you are interested in promoting human rights, whose rights in the breastfeeding relationship take precedence — mother's or baby's? Do either one's rights supersede the other's? Society tends to favor mother's rights over her baby's because baby is a passive participant in the relationship. Babies, however, should be viewed as having a right to breastfeed, not in a sense that obligates the mother legally, but in the sense that no person or group can rightfully interfere with or discourage mother's right to breastfeed her child. While political systems may debate rights, loving families automatically confer full and equal rights leaving no one behind.

You may face even more difficult, more personal paradoxes. Your physician may say he supports breastfeeding, but then push you to consider hormonal contraceptives, which can adversely impact milk supply. Society may interpret "safe" child spacing in a way that contradicts your family's understanding of being open to life.

You, who simply wanted to do what was best for your baby, may find yourself caught unfairly in the midst of these and other contradictions. While there's little you can do to resolve these contradictions or reverse societal attitudes or policies, you can at least educate yourself on the facts (regarding breastfeeding, contraceptive use, amenorrhea, natural child spacing, and natural family planning) so that you and your husband can effectively hedge yourselves against the pressure to abandon breastfeeding before your baby is ready.

Social factors

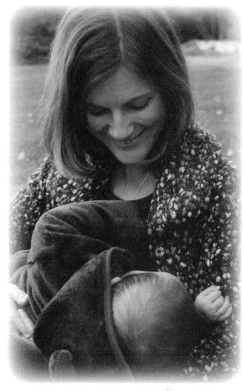

Social influences surround you and demand your attention. Even before you deliver your child, expect pressure to abandon your commitment to breastfeed to come at you from all directions. Social pressures shape our opinions, how we relate to one another and how we view ourselves and our position in the social order. They can be positive or negative. Peer pressure is a powerful social pressure; so are the values passed along by ancestors and our faith traditions. Parents must act in the best interests of their children and their actions should be guided by knowledge, values, spirituality, and heritage. This book is meant to increase your knowledge of breastfeeding *and* lend support for those values that led you to accept the sacrifices required to give and nurture a new life.

Corporate marketers play a role in shaping public opinion and they use money and the media to promote products which they claim to be in a family's best interests. Advertising promotes the idea that manufactured infant formula is not only interchangeable with breast milk, but it is more convenient. If the only benefit your baby reaped from breast milk was nutritional, convenience alone might be a compelling enough reason to reject breastfeeding and use infant formula. Of course, breastfeeding's benefits are far more compelling. Unfortunately, there's no money to be made promoting breast milk.

Media wields a great deal of power too, by choosing what's important or worth reporting, and what isn't. One result has been the elevation of bottle-feeding to a cultural norm while breastfeeding is marginalized as a worthwhile endeavor. The result: those who seek to increase their knowledge and support for breastfeeding end up hearing mixed messages on the value of breastfeeding.

How breastfeeding is portrayed on television leads to a paradox between the need for modesty and the reality of breastfeeding mechanics. Even wholesome family entertainment avoids depicting breastfeeding relationships, which further influences how mothers who breastfeed in public will be accepted. In this way, media doesn't simply reflect society; it influences attitudes.

Other social pressures will be more personal. Adding a baby to your family alters the economics of your household. This change doesn't have to be negative, but many will view it this way. When the size of a family changes, this becomes a good time to examine the family's priorities and accordingly adjust income, work schedules, expenses and outside commitments. Second incomes can sometimes help pay for vacations or other perks, but sometimes second incomes lift a family out of poverty. When taking into account the economic impact of exclusive breastfeeding, you must consider a host of job-related expenses that accompany a second income. When you sacrifice a second income, you also gain back these job-related expenses, which reduce the overall impact to the family budget. Remember, it is up to parents to set their family priorities and shield themselves from external influences that cause them to covet the affluence of others.

The notions of individualism and equality, fundamental American values, are knocked on their heads by breastfeeding. Society, in its quest to equalize the sexes, may recognize the importance of the mother-baby bond, which is facilitated through breastfeeding, but it hasn't been able to reconcile how the art of breastfeeding changes a woman's reality. The supply and demand principle behind successful breastfeeding in reality will remove mother from the many opportunities offered by the marketplace, thereby making it difficult for society to attach a value to her in this new role as nurturer.

Furthermore, the dependence inherent in breastfeeding allows baby to move through his developmental stages at the pace that is right for him. Developmental stages are deliberate and sequential. Mother's presence is more than physical, it is emotional and psychological; in fact, her presence is critical for baby so that he will work his way through his developmental stages properly. Baby's complete dependence on mother early on allows him to mature fully and move toward eventual independence.

Most peoples' experiences are based on formula-feeding. This lack of familiarity with the outcomes of breastfed infants will prompt well-meaning people, possibly including family members, to offer inaccurate assessments of your baby's progress. It can be easy to misjudge what motivates someone to make comments that you perceive as negative. You know breastfeeding fundamentals do not align with formula feeding and you've read research which has revealed the overall health of breastfed babies is better than the overall health of their formula-fed counterparts. Remember this when kindly offering well-meaning detractors new insight and knowledge of the full spectrum of breastfeeding's benefits.

Political considerations

Some wonder what role government should play in promoting breastfeeding. This is a quandary, because few people equate the need to improve breastfeeding initiation rates with increased government regulation. In fact, even the World Health Organization and U.S. government initiatives, which provide breastfeeding guidelines, haven't led to significant increases in breastfeeding continuation rates.

Certainly, the free market can play a role in helping women comfortably breastfeed in public, which can further continuation rates. Many companies offer lounges where mothers can express and store breast milk and some offer on-site daycare where mothers can have access to hungry babies. Some shopping centers have created comfortable spaces for breastfeeding mothers to feed their babies, which allow mothers to get out of the house, get exercise and socialize with others. Other perks enjoyed by new mothers include special parking spots close to building entrances, similar to those available to handicapped patrons. By investing in pleasant public breastfeeding facilities, businesses hope to reap rewards through increased sales and customer loyalty.

It should be considered a positive development when companies come to the realization that supporting breastfeeding is good business. In a perfect world, government intervention shouldn't be required. However, every year we are reminded that not every business or person supports a woman's right to breastfeed in public. In 2006, a breastfeeding mother was asked to leave a commercial airliner prior to take-off because fellow passengers, uncomfortable with her actions, complained to the flight attendant. Her removal led to a firestorm of protests and an apology from the airline.

Women's rights to breastfeed vary from state to state and from place to place. Fourteen states don't have laws protecting women who choose to breastfeed in public; in forty-three states, however, a woman cannot be arrested for indecent exposure because she is breastfeeding in public. In other words, government needs to continue to play a role in protecting women's rights to breastfeed in order for breastfeeding to be considered normal, openly accepted and widely practiced.

Lifestyle adjustments

To achieve breastfeeding success, minor changes to lifestyle may be required. These changes, however, needn't be as negatively perceived as the attitudes reported by the Health Styles 2000 Survey: *Women's Experiences Breastfeeding in Public Places*. This survey sampled attitudes of a cross-section of the United States to reveal that 45 percent of all adults (men and women) felt breastfeeding women had to sacrifice too many lifestyle habits such as favorite foods, smoking, and drinking alcohol. The lifestyle adjustments necessary to accommodate breastfeeding are negligible, however, when factored against breastfeeding's benefits.

Certain beverages, including alcohol, do affect a mother's breast milk. Alcohol gets into a woman's bloodstream in fifteen minutes and into her breast milk in thirty minutes. Even very small amounts of alcohol have deleterious effects on breastfeeding and should be avoided. Alcohol slows the Milk Ejection Reflex; it also causes babies to become sleepy, have difficulty waking, to snore, to have little or no reaction to pain, and for some, affects their ability to suck. Alcohol also decreases milk supply.

To avoid all these effects, it is best to completely avoid alcohol consumption during breastfeeding. Even a glass or two of wine with dinner can be problematic. Mothers who enjoy the taste of beer or wine can find non-alcohol formulations to be a suitable replacement, especially when considering the decision to avoid alcohol is in the best interests of breastfeeding.

Caffeine consumption that exceeds sixteen to twenty ounces per day brings with it risks to a developing fetus. These risks include higher rate of stillbirth, reduced birth weight, accelerated breathing and heart rate after birth, and increased agitation. Caffeine consumption while breastfeeding is generally regarded as safe at lower consumption levels, generally less than sixteen ounces per day. This is not to say baby isn't affected by caffeine. He is. In fact, it may take a newborn two days to eliminate the caffeine from his system. If baby is agitated and isn't sleeping well, evaluate your intake of caffeine from all sources, including coffee, tea, soda, chocolate and even over-the-counter pain relievers and cold medications.

Smoking and exposure to second-hand smoke is harmful to babies; it is known to increase the risk of secondary infections in infants such as respiratory and ear infections. Smoking also decreases prolactin, the hormone necessary for milk production. According to the U.S. Department of Health and Human Services, exposure to smoke has also been associated with an increased risk factor for Sudden Infant Death Syndrome.

The best thing smoking mothers can do for their babies is quit smoking. If quitting is impossible, the government advises women to still breastfeed; better to have babies ingesting nicotine from breast milk than deprive them of all the other benefits of breastfeeding, experts say. However, women should never smoke during a breastfeeding session.

Prescribed and over-the-counter medications could have deleterious effects on breastfeeding and/or baby. If your doctor prescribes a medicine, be sure to ask him to explain all the possible effects the drug may have on milk supply and your breastfeeding child. If you purchase over-the-counter medications, ask for the same information from the pharmacist. Many people self-medicate without consulting a health-care professional; this is an unwise course of action while breastfeeding. If, after consulting with your doctor or pharmacist, you are comfortable with a certain medication's safe use, there are still some ways to minimize its effects. These include:

> ▷ Take oral medications immediately *after* a breast-feeding session.

> ▷ Take oral medications immediately *before* the baby's longest period of sleep.

> ▷ Avoid medications labeled extra strength, maximum strength, or long acting.

> ▷ Use the lowest recommended dose of regular strength products.

> ▷ Avoid combination medications that contain several active ingredients.

Health products using natural herbs are hugely popular and considered by many to fall beyond the scope of "prescribed medications," which can lead to misconceptions about their safety and appropriate use during breastfeeding. The World Health Organization estimates that between 65 percent and 80 percent of the world's population uses herbal medicines as their primary form of healthcare. The following are a few misconceptions regarding the use of herbal products:

HERBAL PRODUCTS TO AVOID DURING BREASTFEEDING	
Aloe vera	Goldenseal
Basil*	Kava Kava
Black Cohosh	Licorice
Bladderwrack	Male fern
Borage	Podophyllum
Buckthorn berry and bark	Purging buckthorn
Colsfoot	Rhubarb Root
Comfrey	Uva Ursi
Ginseng	

*Concern is for therapeutic use, not use as a spice.

Source: International Lactation Consultant Association

> Herbal remedies don't contain pharmacologically active components.

> Herbal remedies are tested and approved by a government agency. (Food sources, including infant formula and some herbal remedies, are categorized as "Generally Regarded As Safe" (GRAS), which means FDA rules for a systematic product assessment regarding safety, effectiveness, standardization or potency, do not apply.)

> Common terms of herbs are accurate representations of the plant that has actually been used in the formulation.

> Usage of herbal remedies does not need to be reported to health care providers when listing medications.

Furthermore, herbal products originating in Third World countries may be contaminated or contain herbs not listed on the label, leading to hidden dangers. Always tell your doctor if you are using herbal remedies while breastfeeding.

The sexuality of breasts

In the United States in the twenty-first century, it has become commonplace to see women's breasts decorated, pierced, tattooed, lifted, branded, augmented or otherwise enhanced for the purpose of making them into objects of sexual attraction. Here is a paradox: Do breasts exist for sexual arousal, or, do they exist to nurture and feed developing infants? Does one purpose automatically exclude the other? Can couples maintain their pre-pregnancy view of breasts during breastfeeding?

Women who become mothers will see themselves expanding… not only physically through pregnancy, but personally. The image of the expanding woman illustrates beautifully what is happening to her; she is *developing* into a more complete, well-rounded individual and this development expands with each pregnancy. As she grows personally, so does her self esteem, her purpose in life and her identity. There is a beauty to be found in describing oneself as a mother and wife. It connotes love and life.

Breasts, also, take on new purpose during this period of growth and development. If a woman previously viewed her breasts as only serving a sexual function, it is likely that she will be embarrassed to use this *sexual object* in public, even for something as worthwhile as breastfeeding. As her view of self and her breasts evolves to include the nurturing component, however, it becomes less difficult to breastfeed publicly. Support from one's husband in this area helps; he is a wife's number one helpmate who (hopefully) assisted her to come to the decision to breastfeed. It is likely he also is expanding and growing in his perception of her breasts.

The female breast, while not a sex organ, is often an enjoyable part of sexual interplay between husband and wife. This doesn't have to change during breastfeeding even though the dynamics of breastfeeding may lead each person to alter their view of the purpose of breasts and how breasts fit into postpartum sexual interplay.

American society is fixated on youth and attractiveness; when breasts are adorned for visual stimulation, both men and women can lose sight of the nurturing purpose of breasts. A woman who chooses to breastfeed might discover societal views of the breast are too narrow or overly-sexualized; society is happy to embrace the sexual nature of her breasts but ignores the nurturing capacity or the ability of breasts to be a primary infant food source. This can result in the creation of tension between men and women as they consider the practice of breastfeeding. Women who understand they are made in the image and likeness of God will be less likely to think of her breasts solely in sexual terms.

Unfortunately, the pursuit of sexually idealized breasts has an effect on breastfeeding rates. In 2001, the number of women who underwent breast augmentation surgery in the United States was 206,354. That represents a 533 percent increase over a ten-year period. In California alone, one out of seven women has undergone breast implant surgery.[1] Rarely is lactation considered when a woman pursues breast augmentation surgery and often her lactation potential is adversely impacted by these procedures.

The narrow societal view of breasts can be reversed, however. Centuries ago, anthropologist Kathyrn Dettwyler tells us, small feet on women were considered by Chinese men to be sexually attractive. The ancient practice of foot binding, however, is today viewed by most as a barbaric practice.

Women will likely choose to breastfeed because of the enormous benefits reaped upon them and their babies. Yet society imposes its attitudes on women leading many, if not most, to feel embarrassed to breastfeed in view of others. Gradually, women can bypass this embarrassment, or at the very least, learn to adjust. This change occurs as a woman's own perception of her body fundamentally aligns with the design of the Creator. The

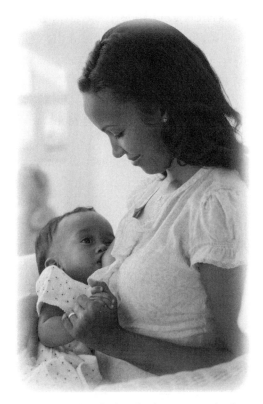

more committed to feeding and nurturing her baby she becomes, the less concerned she'll be over how others view the purpose of breasts. Likewise, breastfeeding couples can and should pass on this new found identity to their children, who will develop a healthy perspective of the purpose of women's breasts. A son who witnesses his mother breastfeeding his siblings will hold a naturally healthier view of the breast, enabling him to support his wife in her decision to exclusively breastfeed. Likewise, a daughter who observes her mother breastfeeding her siblings will see breastfeeding as a natural extension of her femininity and be less self-conscious breastfeeding in sight of others. When the natural purpose of a woman's breast isn't communicated lovingly to sons and daughters as they grow up, culture will define the purpose for them; in the United States, that purpose is primarily sexual.

Few cultures sexualize the mammary glands the way the culture in the United States has. In fact, Dettwyler explains, in most world cultures female breasts are not tied to sexual attractiveness or part of a couples' sexual interplay. Thus, there are significant differences in how humans view the female breast around the world and this variation in attitude drives down breastfeeding rates in countries where breasts help define sexual attractiveness.

Think about how young children in the United States appear on public beaches. Little girls wear swimsuits to cover undeveloped breasts while little boys are free to run around in swim trunks alone. A four-year-old girl running around topless would certainly garner some negative attention. What lessons do little boys and girls learn about breasts from looking at each other over a pile of sand? While we are *not* advocating for four-year-old girls to play topless at the beach, we simply wish to illustrate this point: Cultural attitudes are deeply ingrained in individuals by the time they reach puberty. When you realize how ingrained the sexualization of breasts has become in America, you begin to understand the root of some people's embarrassment seeing, or practicing, breastfeeding in public.

Newcomers to the United States may especially encounter mixed messages regarding the purpose of breasts, which run contrary to views held in their native culture. Assimilation to prevailing cultural mores leads many immigrants to abandon breastfeeding despite having an innate comfort with, and acceptance for, breastfeeding.

The connotation that breasts are sexual objects can skew a woman's own perception of how long to breastfeed according to the gender of her baby. Research reveals that baby boys are typically weaned sooner than baby girls.[2] The reasons are two-fold. First, a mother may perceive a male baby to have a greater energy requirement; this isn't a valid concern because the breasts adjust to each infant's nutritional demands. Plus, complementary feeding (after six months) makes up for any extra calories needed by babies. But more importantly, mother may succumb to psychosocial pressure, i.e., the sexualization of breasts, and often abandon breastfeeding a male baby earlier than she would a baby girl.

Practicing the art of breastfeeding can help the culture de-sensualize the breasts by putting the purpose of a woman's breasts into proper perspective. Understanding cultural attitudes helps explain any embarrassment you or your husband may feel as you initiate breastfeeding and work your way through the process of learning the art of breastfeeding. It's never easy to buck prevailing attitudes, but if you are committed to giving your baby the best possible outcome, it will become easier over time. You will influence the attitudes of those closest to you first then, slowly, others may change their view of breastfeeding because of your commitment to your baby and breastfeeding. Eventually, your circle of influence will expand to help other couples overcome their breastfeeding embarrassment and in your own way, you'll have helped change society for the better.

A historical perspective

In the Victorian era, modesty was stressed and therefore public breastfeeding was discouraged. Furthermore, diseases such as dysentery and cholera forced people to improve upon individual hygiene. Consequently, people viewed bodily fluids, including breast milk, in a negative light. Advertisers took advantage of this shift in perception to push aside breastfeeding in favor of "sterile" rubber nipples and glass bottles to hold manufactured infant formula, which is rarely sterilized. Eventually, breastfeeding began to slip out of the collective consciousness of health-minded Americans.

Industrialization led the medical community, and then parents, to believe babies ought to be regulated and governed according to the clock, much like their factory-working parents. Efficiency in infant care became the gold standard for good mothering. Infants, women were told, were manipulative and could use their screams and tears to wield power over the household. Breastfeeding on demand was believed to lead baby toward self indulgence and a lack of self control, therefore mothers were encouraged to impose schedules on their infants. Even the name given to manufactured infant food — formula — plays to this industrial mindset. It connotes control as the ideal.

Amazingly, some of the rigid mothering principles from the early twentieth century proliferate today, under the guise of offering women freedom from the constraints and demands of breastfeeding. Worries about spoiling babies through frequent breastfeeding may tempt women away from the art of breastfeeding. When this happens, milk supply falls, creating false "insufficient milk syndrome," leading to the perception of failure and ultimately premature cessation of breastfeeding.

Furthermore, during the 1950s, it was widely believed that breastfeeding caused a woman's breasts to droop or sag, playing to a woman's concern over her appearance. Modern research has proven this notion to be untrue, yet the myth persists. Breasts sag for the same reason other body parts sag — age, loss of muscle tone, and excess weight.

The most significant factor contributing to the decline in breastfeeding rates has been the role the medical community has assumed in regulating infant feeding, childbirth, menstruation, and child spacing. As the medical community's interests in women's issues expanded, "control" was touted as an "advancement." The result: many women today allow doctors to influence them on how best to feed their infants and manage reproduction — decisions that, under normal circumstances, can be easily handled by married couples without medical intervention. The consequences for society have been immense. Today, the medical community ignores and even undermines "natural" biological processes in favor of controlling reproduction through chemical or hormonal contraception and childbirth through medicalized procedures. Abortion on demand, artificial conception and unnecessary childbirth interventions, which we learned inhibit breastfeeding success, are all outgrowths of the over-medicalization of naturally-occurring processes.

There are doctors who support breastfeeding and natural family planning and natural childbirth. Local chapters of the Couple to Couple League can be a resource to help you find supportive practitioners in your area. One More Soul is another. (Find contact information for both in Appendix A, at the back of this book.)

Breastfeeding's effects on sexual desire

The intense physical intimacy of the breastfeeding relationship can leave a woman to wonder about the future of her sexual relationship with her husband. The release of oxytocin occurs during breastfeeding *and* during sexual intercourse and produces similar physiological responses and sensations in women's bodies. These responses include: bonding, uterine contractions, and hardening of nipples, all leading to oxytocin being dubbed "the love hormone."

Even though physiological responses to breastfeeding can sometimes mimic sexual experiences, leading to guilt, shame, or confusion in roughly 25 percent of women, the pleasure experienced while breastfeeding is not intrinsically nor biologically *sexual*. Breastfeeding need not lead to a sexual paradox. The pleasure of breastfeeding is indeed natural and facilitates mother-child bonding.

There are issues for breastfeeding couples that will need to be addressed, however, including decreased libido in mother, postpartum discomfort, painful intercourse, changes in the breast such as let-down that often occurs during intercourse, and issues related to fertility. It is important to understand how breastfeeding changes a woman's body and the external factors that can hinder a couple from resuming the sexual relationship they enjoyed prior to baby's arrival.

Libido is sexual drive. Postpartum libido can be affected by many external and internal factors, breastfeeding being just one. Fertility issues, adjusting to a new parenting role, lack of privacy, infant health, pre-existing marital issues, psychological factors unrelated to breastfeeding, attachment issues that interfere with the husband-wife relationship, and/or reduced hormonal activity all can affect how a woman approaches the issue of resuming her sexual relationship.

Emotional attachment between mother and child, which is intense during breastfeeding, can reduce a woman's emotional readiness to connect to her husband as often as she might like. Some studies have revealed that breastfeeding couples engage in sexual intercourse between three and five times per month. Increased maternal age correlated to lower incidence of intercourse while higher incidences were reported among younger women. Not all women will experience changes in their libido after childbirth or during lactation. Some have reported that childbirth and lactation have improved their marital relationship and intimacy.

The natural process of physical recovery from vaginal childbirth takes at least six weeks. New mothers could have tenderness from episiotomies or vulvo-vaginal or perineal stress which may continue for several months.

Studies cited in the *Journal of Human Lactation* report that 62 percent of first-time mothers experience pain upon intercourse during the first three months postpartum. Their numbers drop by half, to 31 percent experiencing pain at six months postpartum. The anticipation of pain associated with postpartum sexual intercourse leaves many women less than enthused about the prospect of resuming sex after childbirth. An added complication for breastfeeding women can be reduced levels of the fertility hormones, which cause extreme vaginal dryness, thinning of the vaginal wall, and reduced production of arousal fluids that lubricate the vagina and help prevent tissue damage during intercourse. The vaginal changes caused by the lack of ovarian activity due to breastfeeding may continue for many months while lactating.

While women's postpartum changes can be physical, they also can be psychological. Many women experience mood changes after childbirth, due to shifting hormones. For some, postpartum depression emerges several days after birth and can last up to several weeks. Such depression affects libido. In addition to hormonal changes comes the added stress that caring for a new infant can place on a woman's energy levels, causing her to view sexual intercourse as just one more responsibility set upon her shoulders.

Exhaustion may be the most pervasive inhibitor of libido. The *Journal of Human Lactation* reports that 25 percent of new mothers indicated tiredness reduced their sex drive. Lactating mothers may be more vulnerable to fatigue than non-lactating mothers, due to the frequency required to maintain adequate milk supply.

During intercourse, breastfeeding mothers may experience let-down, which leads to milk leakage, and for some, embarrassment and discomfort. While fondling lactating breasts has not been found to increase incidences of breast infections or mastitis,[3] tenderness of the breast may cause women discomfort when her breasts are manipulated during foreplay or coitus. When women experience pain or discomfort, their spontaneous non-verbal response communicates the idea that her breasts are now "off limits," affecting libido. A woman's internal response to the natural Milk Ejection Reflex may cause her to conclude it's problematic to include her breasts in sexual foreplay.

First-time fathers may find their perception of their wives changes with lactation. Motherhood and breastfeeding may cause a husband to be more, or less, sexually attracted to his wife. He may fear hurting her or feel guilt over his own sexual desires if he views them as running contrary to her stage of recovery or her new role as nurturer. As a man adjusts to his new role of father, he will undergo psychological shifts which can lead to conflict — or to spiritual awakening and growth. Men must adjust their thoughts, self-image and actions to accommodate the major life event of fatherhood. The application of chastity and periodic abstinence during marriage should allow him to conform to virtuous living. When a man loves his wife as Christ loves the Church, he can sacrifice for the good of his family and not make demands that place his needs above theirs.

New fathers may have a difficult time imagining marriage beyond breastfeeding, which is simply one developmental parenting stage that will give way to others down the road. He will adjust easier if he understands that quality parenting and a loving marriage involve the gift of self and sacrifice.

Breastfeeding's effects on the libido can present temporary and unique challenges to a husband and wife. Therefore, it is important to communicate feelings, goals, needs, and desires while each of you adapt to your new role.

There may be plenty of reasons to want to postpone resuming your sexual relationship. If you resume sexual activity before you are healed for instance, you will experience pain and that will color your future desire to engage in the act of marital love. Any time you anticipate an action is likely to cause pain, you will unconsciously communicate hesitancy, which your spouse may misinterpret as disinterest or a change in feelings. Communication is critical.

With slight exception, factors that either facilitated or inhibited sexual arousal before pregnancy or birth will remain a part of your experience or preference after birth and during breastfeeding. Eventually, normal hormonal activity and cycles will return, eliminating the physiological obstacles caused by the lack of ovarian function during exclusive breastfeeding. This means soon you can, and will want to, resume a sexual relationship with your spouse. A noticeable increase in libido is often a predictor of the return to fertility, the topic covered in chapter seven.

In the early twenty-first century, breastfeeding rates in the United States are highest among highly-educated, upper income women, leading some to look upon breastfeeding as an elitist activity. Ideally, breastfeeding benefits need to be considered outside of socio-economic, political, educational, and even sexual parameters. Breastfeeding benefits baby and mother but also father and society as a whole. It is dangerous to classify breastfeeding as being appropriate only for certain segments of the population. "Breast is best" for everyone.

CHAPTER SIX

Breastfeeding the Older Baby and Baby-led Weaning

At what age does your baby stop being a *baby*? At twelve months? At twenty-four months?

From birth until entering school, children pass through several developmental stages and the labels we use to classify these stages come with social connotations. *Newborn*, *infant* and *baby* connote total dependence on mother while *older baby*, *toddler* and *older child* hint that some level of independence has been achieved.

American culture uses the word *baby* to mean several things. Sometimes it refers to a newborn or infant or very young child; other times, baby refers to the youngest member of the family without regard to age. It also is used to describe a person exhibiting immature or child-like behavior.

Think for a minute how you might define *older baby*. Here's the rub: the definition of older baby varies greatly according to cultural, ethnic, and socio-economic groups. You may even find differing opinions within your own family on what age baby becomes an older baby. Within the art of breastfeeding, older baby is defined as a child older than twelve months of age; this takes into consideration the breastfeeding guidelines set by the American Academy of Pediatrics and the World Health Organization.

While most agree that breastfeeding is best for babies, you might be surprised at how differently the world views breastfeeding an older baby.

Data reported from developing countries reveals that 78 percent of older babies between age twelve months and age fifteen months continue to be breastfed. This is nearly identical to international breastfeeding rates for this age group. By age twenty-four months, that number drops to 45 percent, or less than half of all children in those countries.

In the United States, breastfeeding rates for older babies, measured at age eighteen months, are considerably lower — less than 7 percent. This is a significant deviation from breastfeeding rates found worldwide. What is going on in the United States?

People in the United States seem to want to rush along baby's development, moving him quickly from infanthood to toddlerhood to childhood to adulthood. What is the rush? What considerations might we overlook as we rush to push children through their deliberate and sequential developmental stages, and what might be the consequences?

Breastfeeding provides both nourishment and nurturing regardless of baby's age. These two benefits alternate in importance at different points along the developmental axis of baby's growth. As stated earlier, a woman may start breastfeeding because of its nutritional benefits but continue breastfeeding for others, such as immunological, health, growth, psychological, or social benefits. Older babies encounter many nutritional opportunities beyond the breast. Nutritious supplementary foods, however, cannot provide pain relief, comfort, or security in the way breastfeeding does so beautifully. For example: an older baby who suddenly cannot eat supplementary foods due to illness will find great comfort in the fact that his mother continues to offer nutrition through breastfeeding. During an illness, the older baby breastfeeds primarily to receive nutrition; once illness passes, he breastfeeds for comfort. In other words, mother and older baby still have need to continue breastfeeding and their reasons change according to circumstances.

For older babies experiencing pain, breastfeeding offers analgesic relief, as reported in 2006 in the *International Breastfeeding Journal*: Suckling at the breast stimulates the baby's tactile and oral receptors refocusing attention on the mouth and reducing outside influences. Second, digested fat from breast milk stimulates the release of hormones, which induces relaxation and pain relief. Third, the sweet flavor of milk stimulates the release of opioids in the midbrain of babies, decreasing the perception of pain. Fourth, breastfeeding involves maternal-baby skin to skin contact which helps to stabilize baby's blood glucose, body temperature and respiration, reducing stress and blood pressure.

As older babies grow and thrive through breastfeeding, they often "comfort nurse." Older babies love to breastfeed because of the emotional connection with mother it provides them. The older baby still needs to connect with his mother because his identity remains intertwined with hers. As his identity begins to emerge, he'll begin to explore his world and discover the importance of other people, including his father and other family members. This helps prepare him to wean.

All older babies wean — eventually. The art of breastfeeding allows you to build confidence through breastfeeding; when you master it, you will know your child well enough to understand his needs and be able to meet them while also balancing them against you and your husband's needs, and the responsibilities of your household. By mastering the art of breastfeeding, negative cultural influences will hold little sway in your decision to continue breastfeeding your older baby or at what age it will be appropriate to wean him.

In her book *The Absorbent Mind*, Maria Montessori addresses the topic of child development: "Localized states of maturity must first be established and the effort to force the child's natural development can only do harm. It is nature that directs. Everything depends on her and must obey her commands."

The United Nations Children's Fund points out that breastfed babies generally double their weight by five months, triple their weight by twelve months and quadruple their weight by twenty-four months. During the first six months, babies grow in length an average of one inch per month; between six months and twelve months, growth slows to a half inch per month. Furthermore, a baby's brain increases in size rapidly during early infancy; by age eighteen months, the older baby's brain is 75 percent of the weight of an adult brain. It is important to be aware of these markers because growth rates are the first clue to a baby's nutritional deficiency or suffering.

By the time your baby is four months old, you should have recovered from birthing, your breasts should have adapted to baby's demands, and everything should have reached equilibrium. Around the age of six months, your baby may begin to notice household activities, which can cause him to become distracted or less interested in frequent breastfeeding. This will be the time to consider complementary foods because his growth requires additional vitamins, minerals, proteins, and carbohydrates, things he might not be getting from exclusive breastfeeding.

Breastfeeding can successfully continue for months or even years past the point of introducing complementary foods. Maintaining a balance between continued breastfeeding and complementary feedings is essential to the art of breastfeeding and sometimes difficult to achieve. Complementary foods are not meant to replace breast milk calories or decrease the intensity of breastfeeding. Solid foods do not normally contain the special fatty acids found in human milk which are needed for brain development.

If you offer complementary foods too soon, offer foods at the wrong time, offer the wrong foods or offer the wrong quantity, you displace nutritive calories and breastfeeding will suffer. Breastfeed fully first then offer nutritious complementary foods *only* when baby indicates continued hunger, shown by fussiness.

See Figure 6-1 on pages 113–114 for guidelines on how to introduce solid foods into your baby's diet.

Experts caution against introducing more than one nutritious complementary food at a time and suggest you watch for signs of allergic reactions with each new food item added. Furthermore, it is advisable to use complementary foods in the afternoon and evening so that full breastfeeding in the morning can relieve any possible engorgement you may experience since baby has likely begun to sleep for longer periods during the night.

It is worth noting that there is no evidence that a particular feeding method will guarantee longer nighttime sleep. This is worth remembering as friends or family may encourage introduction of solids before baby is developmentally able to digest them properly.

Signs that baby may be ready for complementary foods include: his ability to sit alone, eruption of teeth, his imitation of proper chewing

FIGURE 6-1. Introducing Solid Foods into a Breastfed Infant's Diet.
Source: Breastfeeding and Human Lactation, 3rd Edition, Jan Riodan, Table 18-5, p530.

When to Introduce	Approximate Total Daily Intake of Solids*	Description of Food and Hints About Giving Them
6–7 months if infant is breastfed	**Dry cereal**: Start with 1/2 tsp (dry measurement); gradually increase to 2—3 tb.	**Cereal**: Offer iron-enriched baby cereal. Begin with single grains. Mix cereal with an equal amount of breast milk.
	Vegetables: Start with 1 tsp; gradually increase to 2 tb.	**Vegetables**: Try a mild-tasting vegetable first (carrots, squash, peas, green beans). Stronger-flavored vegetables (spinach, sweet potatoes) may be tried after infant accepts some mild-tasting ones.
	Fruit: Start with 1 tsp; gradually increase to 2 tb. Divide food among 4 feedings per day (if possible).	**Fruits**: Mashed ripe banana and unsweetened, cooked, bland fruits (apples, peaches, pears) are usually well-liked. Apple juice and grape juice (unsweetened) may be introduced. Initially, dilute juice with an equal amount of water.
		Introduce one new food at a time and offer it several times before trying another new food.
		Give a new food once daily for a day or two; increase to twice daily as the infant begins to enjoy the food. Watch for signs of intolerance.
		Include some foods that are good sources of vitamin C (other than orange juice).
6–7 months if infant is breastfed	**Meat**: Start with 1 tsp and gradually increase to 2 tb. Divide food among 4 feedings per day (if possible).	**Meat**: Offer pureed or milled poultry (chicken or turkey) followed by lean meat (veal, beef); lamb has a stronger flavor and may not be as well-liked initially.
	Dry cereal: Gradually increase up to 4 tb.	Liver is a good source of iron; it may be accepted at the beginning of a meal with a familiar vegetable.
	Fruits and vegetables: Gradually increase up to 3 tb of each.	Continue introducing new cereals, fruits, and vegetables as the infant indicates he is ready to accept them, buy always one at a time; introduce legumes last.

FIGURE 6-1 (continued). Introducing Solid Foods into a Breastfed Infant's Diet.

When to Introduce	Approximate Total Daily Intake of Solids*	Description of Food and Hints About Giving Them
7–9 months if infant is breastfed	*Dry cereal*: Up to 1/2 cup. *Fruits and vegetables*: Up to 1/4 to 1/2 cup of each. *Meats*:Up to 3 tb. Divide food among 4 feedings per day (if possible).	Soft table foods may be introduced—for example, mashed potatoes and squash and small pieces of soft, peeled fruits. Toasted whole grain or enriched bread may be added when the infant begins chewing. If introduction of solids is delayed until now, it is not necessary to use strained fruits and vegetables.
8–12 months if infant is breastfed	*Dry cereal*: Up to 1/2 cup. *Bread*: About 1 slice. *Fruits and vegetables*: Up to 1/2 cup of each. Divide food among 4 feedings per day (if possible).	Continue using *iron-fortified* baby cereals. Table foods cut into small pieces may be added gradually. Start with foods that do not require too much chewing (cooked, cut green beans and carrots, noodles, ground meats, tuna fish, soft cheese, plain yogurt). If fish is offered, check closely to be sure there are no bones in the serving. Mashed, cooked egg yolk and orange juice may be added at about 9 months of age. Sometimes offer peanut butter or thoroughly cooked dried peas and beans in place of meat.

*Some infants do not need or want these amounts of food; some may need a little more food.

and swallowing, his interest in food, or any increase in breastfeeding that does not squelch fussiness.

At age seven months to nine months, breastfeeding accompanied by one or two complementary feedings will normally satisfy baby's daily nutritional needs. As baby nears his first birthday, he'll show an interest in participating in family meals. Do not expect his interest in the family dinner table to automatically signal an imminent end to breastfeeding; normally, he'll still feed often and get most of his calories from breast milk.

By age ten months to twelve months, baby will be fairly mobile — crawling, sitting or standing without assistance, perhaps even walking. He will also have established eating patterns and may turn to mother and breastfeeding for comfort and reassurance more often. It is possible to interpret this increased need for breastfeeding as over-dependence when in fact these behaviors are *developmentally appropriate*. This is normally not a suitable age to consider weaning; in time, older baby will develop to become more independent and signal his readiness to wean.

Each baby will transition from complementary breastfeeding to supplementary breastfeeding differently. When foods begin to replace breastfeeding, the gradual process of weaning has begun.

Why breastfeed an older baby? The benefits for baby

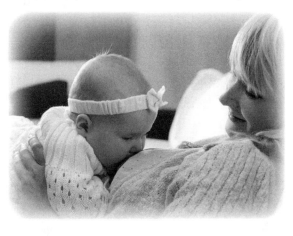

To many people, it seems quite un-natural to continue breastfeeding an old-er baby who is able to drink from a cup and feed himself with a fork and a spoon. Yet there are distinct ad-vantages for mother, baby, and family for continuing to breastfeed the older baby. As stated above, breastfeeding provides relaxation and comfort to older babies. It also provides necessary immunities to augment baby's health, a fact which scientists continue to promote. This is why the World Health Organization encourages breast-feeding to continue to at least age twenty-four months. The composition of human milk changes as baby's feeding patterns change. Immunological factors increase in the breast milk of mothers who breastfeed into the second year offering vital protections to a mobile baby who explores his world hand-to-mouth.

Researchers at the University of California, Berkeley, have linked dura-tion of breastfeeding to reduced risk for two types of childhood leukemia. A 1986 report in *Pediatric Nursing* titled, "The Effects of Breastfeeding on Toddler Health," reviewed the health of breastfed middle class older babies and found a decrease in the number of infections and improved overall health compared to older babies no longer breastfeeding. Other studies show breastfeeding up to age twenty-four months helps prevent diarrhea in the older baby.

Breastfeeding can even have a life-saving dimension during an emergency. In 2006, Kati Kim saved the lives of her daughters (ages seven months and four years) by breastfeeding them while they were stranded in a car during an Oregon blizzard.

Breastfeeding also teaches baby about self-regulation of food intake, an important deterrent to obesity. As you begin to introduce complementary and supplementary feedings, understand that breastfeeding has allowed baby to train himself to recognize when he has had his fill; when he reaches the point of satisfaction, he pulls away from the breast. Your older baby may not be able to pull himself away from the table so easily. It will be up to you to resist the urge to push more food on him than he needs or wants, or require him to finish a portion you have already prepared. High calorie, non-nutritive foods will not satisfy the older baby the way breast milk does and the result may be an older baby who overeats.

Researchers studying participants in the Women, Infants and Children's program offered by the U.S. Department of Agriculture have noted that children between twelve months and age four take in 20 percent to 35 percent more calories than required — leading to childhood obesity concerns. These studies point to consumption of fruit juice and whole cow's milk as contributing factors in excessive weight gain in young children.

Experts have developed nutritional standards for children that begin at age twenty-four months. In the months leading up to this point, it is up to parents to choose and provide to older babies nutritionally optimal food. Given the eight big benefits breast milk and breastfeeding provide, parents interested in giving their children the best possible start in life can be assured that there is a role for continued breastfeeding for their older babies. The years of school lunches, vending machines, fast food restaurants and pre-packaged meals approach quickly enough. Establish good habits early, where baby learns self-regulation and flavor experiences while also enjoying the comfort and reassurance of the maternal bond.

A continued breastfeeding relationship is paramount to raising a happy, healthy child and is fundamental to the art of breastfeeding.

Why breastfeed an older baby? The benefits to mother

Continued breastfeeding benefits mother, both physically and psychologically. For many women, the major advantage of continued breastfeeding is how it promotes emotional well-being. The release of oxytocin, prolactin, and other hormones during breastfeeding reduces maternal anxiety, provides pain relief, reduces mental and physical stress, and lowers blood pressure. Furthermore, breastfeeding mothers have been found to be more socially interactive and are more responsive to their babies; mothers who continue breastfeeding remain sensitive to the needs of the older baby, thereby strengthening the bond that began between them shortly after birth. Continued breastfeeding also helps mothers grow confident as their parenting skills develop in conjunction with baby's developmental growth.

Some consider breastfeeding to be mutual care giving. Continued breastfeeding forces a mother to slow down as she gives her older baby undivided attention several times a day. Through continued breastfeeding, mother relaxes and enjoys time spent with baby while baby gets the nurturing he needs between busy spurts of exploration. It is these daily connections that allow mother and baby to reinforce each other's dignity. Baby's complete dependence upon mother helps her grow in her capacity to care for another human being while her quick response to him instills security that comes from being loved unconditionally.

Breastfeeding babies are generally happy babies. Happy babies make for happy mothers and happy fathers. The result: a happy household. Think about how different society would look if it were filled with happy households!

How social attitudes shape breastfeeding etiquette

With all the benefits babies, women, and families derive through continued breastfeeding, one might think continuation rates would be skyrocketing. Yet earlier you read that while worldwide continued breastfeeding rates hover near 80 percent, American continued breastfeeding rates are less than 8 percent. Some mothers, even those who adamantly support exclusive breastfeeding, have been found to express surprise or even concern about breastfeeding a baby beyond age twelve months. Often, it is the lack of information surrounding the benefits of continued breastfeeding that leads many to wean baby before he is developmentally ready.

Most Americans view breastfeeding as important nutritionally only in the short term. Once complementary foods are introduced, many forget to consider the long term health and emotional benefits accompanying continued breastfeeding. In the wealthiest country in the world where food is abundant, few consider breast milk necessary to the well being of an older baby. Though foods of all types can be found in abundance in the United States, sound nutrition is not a given. Only breast milk contains the humanly manufactured fatty acids essential to brain development and the immunological properties that fight disease.

Furthermore, since fewer than 8 percent of American women breastfeed older babies and few of these women breastfeed in public, Americans are not conditioned to accept breastfeeding for older babies. Breastfeeding occurs in a social context; furthermore, cultural attitudes and beliefs modify American mothers' frequency and duration of breastfeeding. It is very difficult for the unconvinced to breastfeed an older baby when the world expects that child to drink from a cup or bottle. A woman breastfeeding an older baby will undoubtedly receive pressure to wean from someone — her husband, her parents, siblings, friends, coworkers, even other children in the family.

A strategy to achieving success with continued breastfeeding is being prepared for unnerving questions you may receive from others, such as: "How long are you going to nurse?" "Are you *still* breastfeeding?" or "Isn't he getting *too old* to breastfeed?" These disparaging comments can eat away at your resolve to continue practicing the art of breastfeeding.

You can approach this situation two ways. Educate the misinformed on all the benefits you and baby enjoy from breastfeeding. If you are not comfortable defending your personal decisions to others, simply say so,

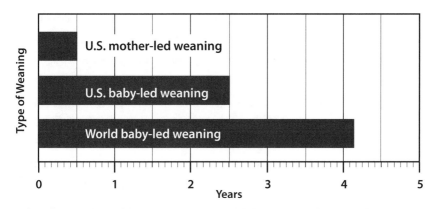

FIGURE 6-2. Average Weaning Ages Throughout World
Source: U.S. Centers for Disease Control.

then use *The Art of Breastfeeding Diary* to journal through some appropriate responses to these questions. Journaling can help you clarify in your own mind the reasons why continued breastfeeding is best for you and your baby, despite others' negative attitudes.

It is well documented that mothers who breastfeed without external pressures will breastfeed for a longer period of time; conversely, mothers with undue societal pressures that view breastfeeding negatively will wean within the first four months. In other cultures, weaning age ranges from twenty-four months to age four. Consider the continued breastfeeding rates found around the world to help you broaden your idea of "normal" as it relates to how you choose to feed and nurture your older baby.

It is not uncommon for parents to feel pressure, or even pressure themselves, to separate from their older breastfeeding baby for an extended period — such as a weekend away. As stated earlier, breastfeeding babies can only tolerate brief periods of separation from mother; this will gradually lengthen throughout his development. Patience and understanding of this developmental need can help both parents set aside a desire to separate from baby, an activity that will threaten continued breastfeeding. Continued breastfeeding does not preclude you from traveling; simply bring baby along and enjoy your family time together.

The art of breastfeeding teaches how important it is to quickly respond to baby's hunger; responding appropriately may have helped you overcome any initial embarrassment you may have felt about feeding in public when it became necessary. First-time mothers soon discover it is easier to breastfeed in public than make baby wait for a more "appropriate" location or time to feed; a screaming baby and soaked clothing from leaking breasts can easily draw more attention to you than feeding baby discreetly wherever you happen to be.

Despite any initial reluctance you might feel breastfeeding in public, you will soon learn what scores of others have discovered about public breastfeeding; as long as you are responding to your baby appropriately, most people will hardly notice what you're doing — or care.

Older babies can accept brief periods of maternal separation, especially during the daytime, when mother is more apt to be out and about. Older babies also will breastfeed less frequently, and will eventually only want to breastfeed first thing in the morning, at naptime, or before bed. This pattern makes it less likely you will need to be concerned with breastfeeding an older baby in public. However, older babies who want to feed at other times but are told they cannot because of activity that takes them into public view can become confused or distressed.

Breastfeeding an older baby in public brings special challenges. Older baby's size and temperament can present difficulties to discreetly breastfeeding in public. Where can you both comfortably sit? What position lends itself to discretion? Will the older baby feed quietly? Is playfulness appropriate? Will the older baby tolerate feeding beneath a blanket? Are there distractions that will prevent successful feeding? The answers to these questions all fall under the topic of breastfeeding etiquette, which relates to baby's feeding conduct, other than suckling.

The art of breastfeeding requires you to follow baby's cues with regard to breastfeeding frequency and intensity; you must, however, mold baby's feeding behavior by setting limits for acceptable conduct. Young babies cry to signal hunger whereas older babies can use language or touch to signal a desire to breastfeed. But which words or touches are appropriate both at home and in public?

Baby must be trained to signal need *and* he must feed in a way that will not embarrass you, cause discomfort, or lead others to view his actions as inappropriate. A twelve-month-old who is not corrected at home for tugging at your blouse or patting your breasts, for instance, will surely repeat this behavior in public. The possible consequence to accommodating such "behaviors" is public embarrassment or scorn, which can cause you to want to wean older baby prematurely.

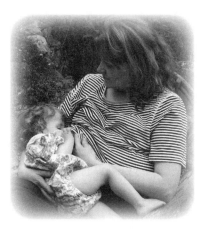

The same is true for breastfeeding positioning and biting. What position has the older baby become accustomed to and does this position lend itself to discreet public breastfeeding? You need to train baby to adapt to a comfortable feeding position that allows for privacy. Does baby use your breast to relieve teething pressure? Suckling and clamping down on the breast cannot occur simultaneously. If baby is biting you during feeding, exercise control over the situation and remove him. Breastfeeding is mutual care-giving but you are the parent; exercise your parental responsibilities and train baby away from habits that interfere with your physical and emotional comfort.

Furthermore, it may be best to teach baby non-verbal signals to indicate his desire to breastfeed rather than having him blurt out embarrassing words such as "milky," "nursey," or "booby." Also, if older baby is easily distracted at the breast while feeding in public, perhaps he can be comforted in other ways. Perhaps offer a nutritious supplemental food and a hug to placate him rather than wrestle with start-and-stop public suckling. Older babies are more adaptable to different situations and will follow mother's instructions regarding breastfeeding etiquette as long as her efforts for effecting change are consistent and meaningful.

Older babies tend to cope with stressful situations by signaling a desire to breastfeed. As babies age, parents must develop a repertoire of appropriate responses to distress, only one of which is breastfeeding. When older babies begin to exhibit coping skills other than automatically turning to breastfeeding, they'll have reached an important marker in the baby-led weaning process. If offers of supplementary foods and alternative comforts fail to console the older baby, it is likely he *really* needs to breastfeed. Recognize that older babies will pass through developmental spurts, meaning their demands for nurturing will occasionally spike.

As the parent, it is incumbent upon you to guide your older baby's behavior and to shape his character with an eye toward virtue. Breastfeeding aids in this goal early on. Breastfeeding behaviors are learned — even those that make you uncomfortable. It is important not to tolerate habits which make you want to prematurely wean your older baby. Set the parameters for breastfeeding behavior early and keep him in check consistently.

Weaning

Weaning is the process of gradually or suddenly transferring baby's dependence on breast milk to another form of nourishment. The process often begins as baby is introduced to supplementary foods, which replaces breast milk calories. At some point, all of a baby's calories will come from supplementary foods and he will lose interest in breast milk. When this process occurs at baby's own pace, it is called baby-led weaning. The art of breastfeeding encourages baby-led weaning.

In some circumstances, a mother will stop breastfeeding before receiving cues that baby is ready. Her reasons may vary from health-related to social or economic pressures. Whatever the reason, when mother initiates the end of breastfeeding, this is called mother-led weaning.

When breastfeeding ceases, milk synthesis normally stops as well, although the process of milk dry-up varies from woman to woman and can last several weeks. (If milk secretions continue beyond one year after weaning, medical intervention should be sought.) Remarkably, the consistency of breast milk at the end of the breastfeeding continuum resembles colostrum, the earliest milk secreted after childbirth.

During the first year of life, a baby will pass through several stages where he may exhibit decreased interest in breastfeeding. These time periods occur around four months to five months, again at seven months, and again between nine months and twelve months. Often, this lack of interest in breastfeeding is the result of some external stimuli. A baby who loses interest in breastfeeding early (during his first year) can be nudged back into breastfeeding by mother. It is up to each woman to decide if reversing these early tendencies toward baby-led weaning is appropriate, keeping in mind the benefits both baby and mother reap while practicing the art of breastfeeding.

Most babies, however, will not lose complete and permanent interest in breastfeeding until after age twenty-four months. The key to successful baby-led weaning is to breastfeed only when baby indicates a need while also providing him with sufficient nutrition through healthy supplemental foods. This is a gradual process by which baby may offer the following clues to his intention to wean:

> ▷ Baby is content and displays increasing independence.

> ▷ Baby shows a greater interest in supplementary solids and liquids, and prefers taking meals at the family table.

> ▷ Breastfeeding frequency and intensity is greatly diminished.

> ▷ Baby is easily distracted at the breast, shows disinterest, or refuses the breast.

Baby-led weaning is a fundamental stage in a child's development, illustrating increased awareness of himself, his world and his place in the family. Weaning is maturation. It is a significant milestone in your relationship, just like the day he was born, the day he took his first steps, the day he said his first word.

Mother-led weaning, while sometimes unavoidable, can lead to problems because it normally occurs much more rapidly than baby-led weaning. Fast-paced mother-led weaning can prevent mother and baby from physiologically and emotionally adapting to such a significant change. There can be a shift in how a mother nurtures a baby post-weaning and this change can cause baby to become more demanding or needy. Baby can also experience stomach upset, constipation or allergic reactions due to his change in diet. Furthermore, baby's health may be compromised because he no longer receives immunity protection specific to breast milk.

Fast-paced mother-led weaning can cause a woman's breasts to become uncomfortably engorged and she will have to express milk to relieve this discomfort.

Mother-led weaning is best done gradually to minimize its effects on both mother and baby.

While some emergency situations may lead to mother-led weaning, they do not have to. If a baby is ill and unable to breastfeed for an extended period of time, a woman can maintain her milk supply by using an electric breast pump, which best imitates baby's sucking action. (Manual pumps are much less effective at emptying the breast for purposes of maintaining milk supply.) If mother is ill or hospitalized for an extended period, it still may be possible for her to maintain milk supply during her separation from baby. Breastfeeding offers many benefits to mothers and babies — even during illnesses; contact a lactation consultant or your health care provider for guidance on how to maintain the breastfeeding relationship during a health care emergency.

Throughout history, researchers have attempted to discover the "magic" age for when to introduce solid foods and wean a baby from the breast. In 1953, one physician developed a regimen of introducing solids to infants on the second day of life. In 1473, one German physician withheld all solid foods until baby had sufficient teeth to chew thoroughly. Other scientists have suggested a weaning date based on weight measurements, calculating birth weight to average adult weight or present weight to birth weight.

Despite the attempts of scientists and physicians to pinpoint the "perfect" age to wean your baby, such a date cannot be predicted. The beauty of the art of breastfeeding comes through the mutual care-giving relationship you have developed as you learn baby's cues and respond to them appropriately.

Practicing the art of breastfeeding during the weaning stage can be difficult if baby shows a readiness to wean and you do not. As baby matures, he grows more independent and his universe expands to include his father, siblings, friends, and relatives. The presence of others in your baby's life in no way diminishes your importance to him. Sure, he is relying less and less on breastfeeding for nutrition and nurturing, but he still needs you as you begin to share him with the world. Weaning, therefore, is an important developmental stage in both of your lives.

CHAPTER SEVEN

The Return of Fertility

As you learn and practice the art of breastfeeding, you may begin to wonder when, if, how, and even why fertility ceases during one part of lactation and returns during another. Women who exclusively breastfeed a first child may be surprised, or even concerned, when their monthly menstrual cycles do not return for months after childbirth. Even women who practice mixed breastfeeding may find their return to fertility is delayed or otherwise impacted by breastfeeding. Childbirth, and certainly breastfeeding, alters the reproductive system in ways that can be confusing and, for some, concerning. What is happening to you? Your reproductive system is in transition as a result of childbirth; furthermore, breastfeeding extends this transition state, depending upon how you feed.

Lactational amenorrhea is a completely normal phenomenon and is defined as the absence of menstruation due to the continual production and removal of mother's milk. The process by which lactation inhibits ovulation and its accompanying menstruation is complex and not completely understood, but in large part is directly tied to hormones secreted due to milk synthesis.

Prolactin, the hormone secreted as a result of baby's feeding and tied to the delay of ovulation, rises after each breastfeeding session and falls sometime thereafter. High prolactin levels inhibit increased estrogen production which is necessary for ovulation and menses. Furthermore, the level of prolactin is directly related to the frequency, intensity, and

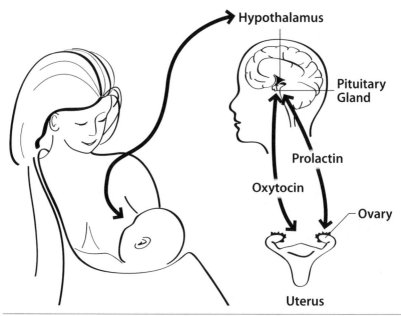

FIGURE 7-1. Hormonal Influences on Lactactional Amenorrhea
Source: Modified from *Breastfeeding and Human Lactation*, 3rd edition, Jan Riodan, Figure A.02.

duration of nipple stimulation due to breastfeeding. When more than eight breastfeeding sessions continue to occur in a twenty-four hour period (exceeding 120 minutes), prolactin levels remain at a concentrated level high enough to normally suppress ovulation. If a woman does not breastfeed, prolactin levels drop to pre-pregnancy levels by seven days postpartum.

Other factors shown to affect the length of a woman's lactational amenorrhea include: time between birth and first feeding; the number of previous births; the frequency and length of breastfeeding sessions; timing of complementary feedings; mother/baby schedules; proximity to baby; employment status; circumstances surrounding initiating breast-feeding immediately after childbirth; the frequency of night feedings; and mother's age, body mass index, and health.

In chapter one, we introduced several terms related to breastfeeding: exclusive breastfeeding, mixed breastfeeding, continued breastfeeding, complementary feeding, and supplementary feeding. Up to this point, this nomenclature described breastfeeding behavior. When explaining breast-feeding's effect on fertility, it is necessary to bring forward additional, more precise terminology and a brief description of the reproductive process to further help you understand what goes on during this "transition state," which along with premenopause, is one of two significant transitions a woman can experience during her reproductive life.

Terms related to fertility

Basal body temperature. Temperature of the body after a night's sleep, which is unaffected by food, drink or activity.

Breakthrough bleeding. Flow of blood from the uterus not preceded by ovulation.

Circadian Rhythm: This normal rise and subsequent fall in body temperature is known as the circadian rhythm. Body temperature rises during the early morning hours and begins to fall in the evening. Basal thermometers measure the temperature of the rested body unaffected by drink, food or activity at the same time within this circadian rhythm.

Fertility cycle. A woman's reproductive cycle can be divided into three phases. *Phase I* relates to the infertile period of time from onset of menses until the first day of fertility. *Phase II* is the stage of fertility when pregnancy can be achieved. *Phase III* is another infertile period of time following ovulation and ending with the onset of menses.

Follicle. Clusters of cells in the ovary capable of producing hormones; when properly stimulated, will release an ovum or egg.

Hormones. Chemical signals produced by the body necessary to maintain cellular activity. Primary hormones affecting fertility cycles include: insulin, progesterone, estrogen, luteinizing hormone (LH), follicle stimulating hormone (FSH), prolactin and oxytocin.

Luteal phase. All days of elevated basal body temperatures following ovulation up to the first day of menstruation in the next cycle.

Menses. Periodic flow of blood from the uterus after ovulation.

Ovulation. Release of an ovum, or female egg, from the ovary.

Pituitary-ovarian axis. A two-way communication system between the brain and the ovaries, which coordinates the timing of ovulation, the production of hormones, and either the maintenance of a pregnancy or the onset of a menstrual period.

What is happening to my body?

The art of breastfeeding is a personal commitment to meeting the unique needs of your infant. It is not a prescription for how often or how long to breastfeed nor is it a method of Natural Family Planning (fertility awareness). The art of breastfeeding is learning to recognize and respond to baby's emotional and physical needs.

Studies on breastfeeding do offer insight into the factors which can affect the length and variability of lactational amenorrhea; this break from cycling and fertility is considered by many to be a benefit of breastfeeding.[1]

Researchers working with the World Health Organization lumped factors affecting amenorrhea into two categories: variables related to breastfeeding and variables not related to breastfeeding. More than eighty-three variables within both categories were analyzed for their impact on the length of amenorrhea; of those, roughly 10 percent were considered significant. As you examine the factors that can affect the length of amenorrhea, understand that averages presume similarities that may not exist in your situation.

Factors that can affect the duration of lactational amenorrhea

No two women will have identical combinations of breastfeeding and non-breastfeeding variables affecting lactational amenorrhea; therefore, one woman's amenorrhea may not resemble another woman's experience. A precise formula for predicting the length of lactational amenorrhea is not possible at this time, although the following variables have been reported to affect the duration of amenorrhea:

Non-breastfeeding variables affecting lactational amenorrhea

1. Shorter periods of amenorrhea are seen in women who have high body mass indices and longer periods of amenorrhea are associated with women who have lower body mass indices. (BMI was measured at six-weeks and eight-weeks postpartum.)

2. Shorter amenorrhea is associated with mother's advancing age.

3. Longer amenorrhea is associated with women who frequently seek out medical intervention for ill babies or whose babies have lengthy illnesses.

4. Pregnancy hormones are variable for each pregnancy and for each woman.

Breastfeeding variables affecting lactational amenorrhea

1. Shorter amenorrhea is associated with delayed initiation of breastfeeding after delivery. For mothers who breastfed within ten minutes of birth, the mean duration of amenorrhea was 182 days; mothers who delay initiation of breastfeeding for four to six hours after birth average seventy-seven days of amenorrhea.

2. Shorter amenorrhea is associated with early (prior to six months) introduction of supplementary food or drink. Decreased suckling at the breast decreases the length of lactational amenorrhea.

3. Shorter amenorrhea is associated with infant's use of a pacifier. The most common consequence to pacifier use is postponing feeding which reduces frequency. Pacifiers often are introduced during the first month, a critical period in which to establish adequate milk supply. Research shows that exclusively breastfed infants who use a pacifier breastfeed at least one less session per day than infants who aren't offered

---

EXPLAINING BODY MASS INDEX

Body Mass Index (BMI) is a formula that uses weight-to-height ratio to estimate your body fat and health risks. A BMI between 18.5 and 24.9, is considered healthy. A person with a BMI between 25 and 29.9, is considered overweight. When a BMI is higher than 30, the person is considered obese.

Healthy: 18.5-24.9
Overweight: 25-29.9
Obese: Higher than 30

Source: BMI calculator: http://www.mayoclinic.com/health/bmi-calculator/nu00597

a pacifier. One less feeding per twenty-four hour period can reduce the length of postpartum amenorrhea.

4. Shorter amenorrhea is associated with mother's return to employment.[3]

5. Shorter amenorrhea is associated with fewer than eight breastfeeding sessions in a twenty-four hour period. Studies indicate that mothers who practice exclusive breastfeeding normally feed baby between twelve and fourteen times (120-140 minutes) per twenty-four hour period, including several nighttime feedings.

6. Longer amenorrhea is associated with greater than 180 breastfeeding minutes in a twenty-four hour period.[2]

7. Longer amenorrhea is associated with exclusive breastfeeding for the first six months. Complementary feeding in which baby is breastfed first and there are no decreases in breastfeeding patterns does not appear to decrease amenorrhea provided such feeding occurs after age six months.

8. Longer amenorrhea is associated with high breastfeeding frequency, high milk volume, intensity of suck, and longer feeding sessions both day and night. Shorter intervals between sucking episodes is associated with longer amenorrhea.

9. Longer amenorrhea is associated with more frequent night feedings. Prolactin is released in higher concentrations during night feedings than during daytime feedings.

10. Previous breastfeeding experience is the greatest predictor of return to fertility.

As you can see, there is a direct correlation between the frequency of breastfeeding sessions and the duration of lactational amenorrhea. Still, it is important to recognize that an average is just that; your experience may or may not fit the patterns outlined above. Your goal is to learn and practice the art of breastfeeding for doing so will provide you and your baby a host of benefits, only one of which may be lactational amenorrhea.

Other facts about lactational amenorrhea worth noting include:

▷ For women practicing mixed breastfeeding, the earliest recorded menses occurred between four and six weeks postpartum.[4]

▷ During lactational amenorrhea, studies reveal that many women experience a "first bleed" or warning period prior to the first ovulation. However, the longer her amenorrhea, the *greater* the likelihood that ovulation will occur *before* the first menses.

▷ Any fertility signs or first bleeds indicate that amenorrhea is nearing an end.

▷ The earlier a first ovulation occurs, the less likely it is characterized by a luteal phase of adequate duration necessary to support pregnancy. Some studies point to continued suckling and consequent elevated prolactin as the cause for inadequate luteal function in the first cycles postpartum.

▷ Mucus patches commonly begin to appear two months prior to first menses.[5]

▷ Cigarette smoking causes prolactin levels to drop.

▷ Topical anesthetics applied to nipples (for soreness) hinder prolactin surges during suckling.

▷ Tandem feeding (two babies simultaneously) doubles prolactin surges.

Results from multiple studies conducted in numerous countries were compiled at the Bellagio Consensus Conference and published in 1988. The conclusions which emerged from this conference offered significant insight into breastfeeding's impact on a woman's fertility during the first six months postpartum. Its conclusions reaffirm the belief that a mother who is exclusively breastfeeding and who remains free of menses (amenorrhic) has only a 2 percent probability to achieve pregnancy prior to six months postpartum. Furthermore, the conference acknowledged that the intensity of exclusive breastfeeding creates physiologic conditions causing a warning period prior to a woman's first adequate ovulation. **These conclusions are only valid for exclusive breastfeeding.**

The Bellagio Consensus Conference generated international interest in expanding the study of how long women can remain infertile while relying on exclusive and continued breastfeeding to space pregnancies; in fact, studies within the conference showed that women who exclusively breastfed for the first six months had a mean average of 7.1 to 15.2 months of lactational amenorrhea.[6]

Since the intensity of mixed breastfeeding varies, the patterns were divided into these sub-categories: high-mixed, medium-mixed, and low-mixed. High-mixed means more than 80 percent of the baby's nutrition is derived from breast milk or breastfeeding. Medium-mixed means between 20 percent and 79 percent of baby's nutrition is derived from breast milk or breastfeeding. Low-mixed means that less than 20 percent of infant's nutrition comes from breast milk or breastfeeding. The suckling that takes place with mixed breastfeeding may be sufficient enough to suppress ovulation, yet not frequent or strong enough to inhibit hormones necessary for production of fertile mucus. The result: women who practice mixed breastfeeding ought to expect heightened ambiguity as they analyze their fertility clues during the transition state. Here, more than ever, understanding your signs and Natural Family Planning's transition rules are keys to effectively managing your returning fertility.

Is breastfeeding an effective way to space babies?

Uncertainty over whether fertility's return is imminent and outside pressure can cause couples who are not ready for pregnancy to fear their returning fertility and turn to hormonal birth control methods. There is no adequate evidence to prove using hormonal contraceptives while breastfeeding is safe for baby and will not impede milk production. Despite conflicting information circulating around the medical community on the safe use of hormonal contraceptives while breastfeeding, prudence demands that women not ingest any substance that can hinder the quality and quantity of breast milk. Furthermore, hormonal contraceptives are considered an affront to human dignity because they alter a healthy, major functioning system of the body, becoming an impediment to loving according to the creative intention of God. (See *The Art of Natural Family Planning® Student Guide*, published by the Couple to Couple League, for a more complete discussion of behaviors that attack human dignity and marital love.)

Despite what we know about fertility status while breastfeeding, the medical community maintains a negative outlook on the effectiveness of natural approaches to fertility management afforded to women who exclusively breastfeed. Many physicians promote breastfeeding as "best for baby," yet deny the proven effectiveness of lactational amenorrhea combined with Natural Family Planning as a way to effectively space pregnancies. Instead, they offer artificial processes and position them as safe so that breastfeeding rates increase.

Recently, the American College of Obstetricians and Gynecologists (ACOG) stated: "Breastfeeding and child spacing are not mutually exclusive if mother uses contraception. If a breastfeeding woman needs or wants more protection from pregnancy, options are available that do not affect breastfeeding or pose even a theoretical risk to the infant. First, she should consider non-hormonal methods."[7] If no *theoretical* risk to using hormonal contraceptives while breastfeeding exists, why does the ACOG suggest women first consider non-hormonal methods, especially early in the transition state?

The Academy of Breastfeeding Medicine (ABM) cautions women away from hormonal contraceptives because their use affects lactation, especially when women have had a history of lactation failure, breast surgery, are breastfeeding multiples, are breastfeeding a pre-term infant, or if her or her baby's health is compromised.[8] When ranking fertility management methods, the ABM suggests Natural Family Planning as a first choice over less suitable hormonal contraceptives.

Many couples are able to effectively rely on lactational amenorrhea to sufficiently space pregnancies according to their family's needs. Other couples experience the return to fertility before they are ready to again achieve pregnancy. These couples can rely on the signs of fertility readily apparent during the transition back to full ovarian function. These signs

— mucus and cervical changes (including basal body temperatures) — are the result of prolactin decreases and estrogen increases. They constitute the basis for Natural Family Planning.

Although an explanation of the signs used in Natural Family Planning is offered below, comprehensive education in Natural Family Planning, including NFP during the postpartum transition state, is recommended and is available through the Couple to Couple League. CCL's postpartum class is designed to specifically address and explain the fertility signs you observe while breastfeeding and can help you successfully use Natural Family Planning during the transition state. Natural Family Planning and breastfeeding do indeed complement one another.

In summary, lactating mothers are normally afforded a significantly longer rest and recovery period before being able to achieve subsequent pregnancy. Exclusive breastfeeding provides the optimum infant nutrition along with a host of other benefits while also offering many couples a child spacing effect that can last for months. Yet even if breastfeeding does not produce lengthy amenorrhea, it is still best for babies, mothers, fathers, and society.

How fertility cycles work

Normal fertility cycles allow couples the opportunity, under most circumstances, to achieve pregnancy. Each fertility cycle brings with it the potential for achieving pregnancy if couples have marital relations during the fertile phase. The process begins with the pituitary gland, which secretes hormones such as follicle stimulating hormone (FSH) that initiates follicular development in the ovaries. Continued follicular growth requires additional FSH *and* estrogen *and* luteinizing hormone (LH). When hormones are in proper balance, ovulation occurs.

Estrogen produces cervical mucus, facilitating fertility. It also softens, raises and opens the cervix, signaling approaching fertility. Under the influence of rising estrogen, cervical mucus secretions become increasingly "more-fertile," producing the sensations of wetness and slipperiness along with a stretchy characteristic. Any mucus is a sign of fertility but this "fertile mucus" signals a closer proximity to ovulation than less-fertile mucus.

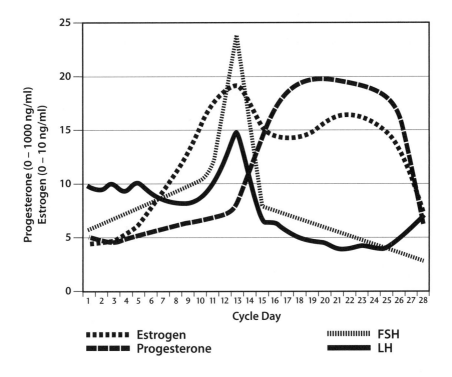

FIGURE 7-2. Relative Hormone Levels During Regular Cycles
Source: Modified from *The Art of Natural Family Planning Student Guide*, Relative Levels of Estrogen and Progesterone, p17; FSH and LH Levels, p18.

The follicle from which the ovum is released transforms into a structure called the *corpus luteum*, producing progesterone which signals the pituitary gland to stop additional follicular development for the remainder of this cycle. While the ovum travels from the ovary to the uterus via the fallopian tube, fertilization may be possible if the husband's sperm (male reproductive cells) are present. Each male ejaculation can yield between 200 million and 500 million sperm cells. When an egg becomes fertilized, it travels from the fallopian tube into the uterus where it attempts to implant. Life begins at conception and follows a continuum of developmental changes that continues through implantation, fetal development, birth, and beyond.

Following ovulation, a woman enters the final phase of her menstrual cycle. It is a time of infertility and typically accounts for the last one-third of a healthy cycle. This part of the cycle is generally constant in length from cycle to cycle. It is noted by an accompanying rise in basal body temperature, due to the post-ovulation release of the hormone progesterone. If pregnancy does not occur, menses follows ovulation by approximately two weeks. At this time, the basal body temperature drops to its pre-ovulatory level. The start of menses essentially marks the beginning of a new cycle; it is the first day of the next cycle, when the process begins anew. Rhythmicity, as seen in fertility cycles, is a normal characteristic of all living organisms. Couples can easily take note of their natural rhythms, chart their observations, identify the fertile and infertile times of their cycles, and use them to plan their families accordingly. This knowledge is known as Natural Family Planning.

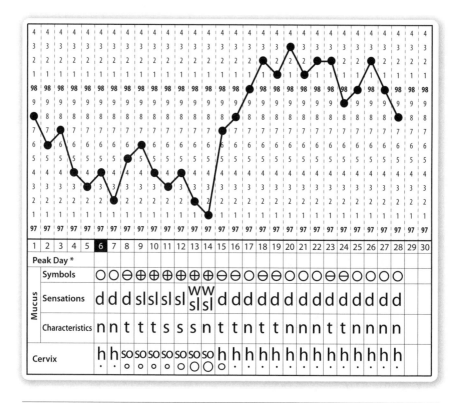

FIGURE 7-3. A Normal Fertility Cycle
Source: Modified from *The Art of Natural Family Planning® Student Guide*, p189.

The postpartum reproductive cycle: a transition state

The production and maintenance of high levels of prolactin brought on through exclusive breastfeeding brings about changes to a woman's fertility and monthly cycles in the months after childbirth; as stated earlier, the pathways between lactation and the suppression of ovulation are intermingled in complex ways.

What is known is that breastfeeding affects the normal reproductive process in this way: Nipple stimulation leads to the secretion of prolactin and other hormones necessary for lactation while also suppressing fertility hormones necessary for ovulation. Without regular and adequate stimulation of the ovaries, fertility cycles are not possible. In other words, exclusive breastfeeding normally can bring about an extended period of natural infertility due to inadequate ovarian stimulation. The length of lactational amenorrhea varies from woman to woman, but is normally longer than six months while practicing exclusive and continued breastfeeding.

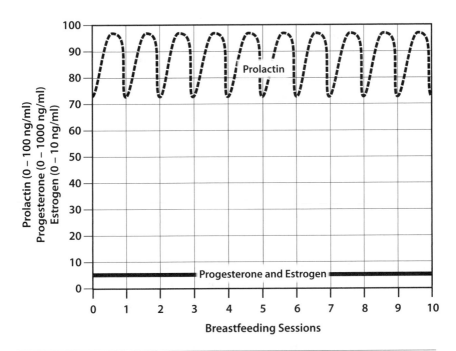

FIGURE 7-4. Relative Hormone Levels During Breastfeeding Amenorrhea
Source: *Breastfeeding: A Guide to the Medical Profession.*

Women who do not breastfeed at all will return to their pre-pregnancy fertility much sooner than lactating women; women who practice mixed-breastfeeding will likely return to fertility sooner than women who practice exclusive and/or continued breastfeeding.

Lactogenesis (initiation of milk secretion) is actually part of the transition state, which begins soon after pregnancy was achieved and will continue until baby weans. As long as regular and continual milk production and removal is underway, several hormonal factors combine to alter one's previously "normal" fertility cycles creating a transition state. The hormonal effect of lactation on fertility cycles includes: amenorrhea, longer cycles, shorter luteal phases, irregular cycles, and altered mucus and/or cervix signs.

For women who exclusively breastfeed during the first six months and continue to breastfeed thereafter, the return to normal ovarian function and the gradual return to fertility after childbirth passes through identifiable sequences. It begins with full but natural infertility with a noticeable absence of cervical mucus secretions, vaginal dryness, and absence of menses. The cervix is low, firm and closed but in a different way than before birthing stretched the cervical muscle. There will be a corresponding low and irregular basal body temperature.

As mucus secretions recommence, their appearance will be sporadic and brief. The mucus that is produced first is usually tacky and does not stretch easily; instead it tends to break when pulled apart. Women have described it as sticky, thick, pasty, creamy, clumpy or having some stretch, but thicker than the more-fertile type of mucus. As estrogen levels begin to rise, a consequence of decreased prolactin, which is itself likely the result of decreased breastfeeding activity, cervical mucus secretions increase in quantity, quality, and frequency. When this type of mucus is present in normal fertility cycles, pregnancy can occur.

As estrogen levels rise, cervical mucus can be felt or sensed. The high estrogen levels around the time of ovulation can thin or liquefy the mucus so much that it literally runs out of the vagina. Many women will experience a strong feeling or sensation of wetness and/or slipperiness when wiping. In fact, sometimes no mucus is visible at all and women just sense a strong feeling of wetness. The sequencing of mucus secretions alternating with dry patches is different from the sequencing of mucus experienced during regular (non-lactating) cycling because during lactation, mucus can appear and disappear without an accompanying ovulation.

Another clue to the return of fertility is first menses. When postpartum discharge has stopped and scanty bleeding occurs before fifty-six days postpartum, this bleeding can normally be ignored as a sign of fertility when exclusively breastfeeding. Some women will experience a "warning" period prior to the return to fertility. This may or may not have been preceded by mucus signs. Experiencing a warning period presumes fertility cycles are resuming.

If there is a desire to postpone another pregnancy, any signs of potential returning fertility should be accompanied by abstinence until the post-ovulation infertile phase is reached. Elevated basal temperatures establish the "luteal" phase and predict the onset of menses. Expect luteal phases in the first few post-amenorrhea cycles to be shorter than normal but to gradually lengthen over time. Once ovulation occurs, menses follows if pregnancy is not achieved.

Short luteal phases are an indicator of temporary infertile cycles as the uterus may not be sufficiently prepared to host a developing embryo. As you approach the end of the transition state (weaning), overall cycle lengths will shorten, luteal phases will lengthen, and cycle irregularities will diminish until they resemble your pre-pregnancy pattern. The pace by which a woman passes through these stages varies greatly from woman to woman due to many of the factors outlined in this chapter.

(For a comprehensive explanation on fertility awareness and NFP, refer to *The Art of Natural Family Planning*® *Student Guide*, published by The Couple to Couple League.)

When do I observe fertility signs while breastfeeding?

Non-lactating women and low-mixed breastfeeders practicing Natural Family Planning need to begin fertility observations and recording of body temperatures by three weeks postpartum due to the likely early return of fertility.

Medium-mixed breastfeeders would be wise to follow the charting guidelines for low-mixed feeders unless prior personal experience indicates prolonged amenorrhea and/or a later return of fertility should be expected.

High-mixed feeders, who remain amenorrheic and free from the presence of fertility signs will not have to chart until six months postpartum or later unless they observe fertility signs or have had previous experience that indicates fertility may return earlier. Once any of the signs of fertility occur, i.e. mucus, cervix changes, or bleeding, charting must begin immediately. These guidelines assume a minimum of eight or more feeding sessions (120 minutes) per twenty-four hour period. The introduction of solids, even prior to six months, increases the likelihood of an early return of fertility, therefore the charting of fertility signs is advisable.

It is not unusual for exclusive breastfeeders to not need to begin charting observations until nine months postpartum, unless their fertility signs, bleeding, or previous experience indicates an earlier return to fertility. Exclusive breastfeeding offers mothers the longest period of lactational amenorrhea.

Use *The Art of Breastfeeding Diary* to note daily, weekly, and monthly breastfeeding activity, such as feeding frequency, supplementary feedings, night feedings, cervical and mucus observations, etc. Also, it is recommended to attend CCL's postpartum transition class for adequate instruction.

The transitional state of fertility brought about by pregnancy, childbirth, and lactation, offers women opportunities and challenges. The reproductive system's response to lactation offers insight into the intricacy and beauty of God's design, something that should comfort us, not fill us with anxiety or fear.

When does the body return to normal?

Contrary to popular belief, women who breastfeed return to their physical pre-pregnancy state sooner than women who do not breastfeed — excepting, of course, her lactating breasts and her fertility cycles. As we explained in chapter three, breast development begins for women *in utero*

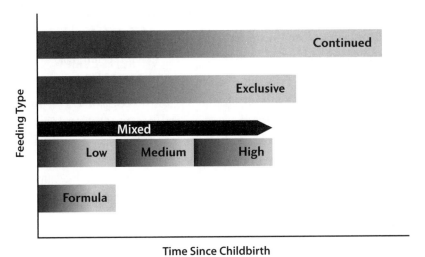

FIGURE 7-5. Relative Return of Fertility
Source: *The Art of Natural Family Planning® Student Guide*, Relative Return of Fertility, p160.

and continues until roughly age thirty-five. Women's fertility cycles begin in puberty and continue — interrupted only by pregnancy and lactation — until menopause, which should be expected around age fifty.

It is not unusual for some women to experience nine months or longer of lactational amenorrhea. A variety of different lactation studies show that early introduction of supplementary feedings along with reduced frequency and intensity of breastfeeding (due to the use of schedules, pacifiers, or skipped night feedings) reduces the duration of natural lactational amenorrhea. Frequent suckling at the breast is necessary for meeting both the physical and emotional needs of your baby and is necessary for maintaining adequate milk supply. Frequent suckling also serves to postpone ovarian and menstrual activity due to the increased secretion of prolactin, the same hormone necessary for milk production. Therefore, the actions and reactions within breastfeeding are multidirectional and provide many benefits: frequent suckling satisfies baby's physical and emotional needs while maintaining sufficient milk supply; it also benefits mothers by helping them heal from childbirth and by providing a natural respite from menses, fertility cycles, and possible pregnancy, a benefit they normally enjoy for more months than their non-lactating sisters.

Of course, there may be exceptions to lactation's cause-and-effect on fertility. Some exclusive breastfeeding mothers may experience an early return to full ovarian function while other mixed breastfeeding mothers may experience prolonged amenorrhea. Some mothers who wish to conceive may be unable to achieve pregnancy until after full weaning, despite cycling that includes ovulation and menses. Yet other women who provide limited infant nutrition through breastfeeding may experience amenorrhea or irregularity. Experiences such as these occur rarely but need to be noted as a reminder that each woman experiences the return of fertility uniquely.

For first-time mothers, the introduction of solid foods may be the strongest predictor of fertility's return. For women who are repeating the breastfeeding experience, the greatest predictor of fertility's return will be her previous experience. Even though each woman is unique and therefore no scientist, doctor, or author can predict how soon fertility will return postpartum, a woman can confidently observe and interpret her individual fertility clues knowing that previous experience will likely repeat under normal conditions.

LEAGUE TEACHES HOW TO APPLY NFP RULES DURING BREASTFEEDING

The Couple to Couple League, a promoter and teacher of Natural Family Planning since 1971, has developed a postpartum Natural Family Planning class that specifically addresses how to detect the return of fertility during this transition state. If you haven't attended this CCL postpartum transition class or the full Natural Family Planning series, contact your local CCL chapter or look online at www.ccli.org for a class near you. Home study courses are available.

For women not in the transition state, Natural Family Planning is 99 percent effective. Lactation introduces variability and ambiguity to reemerging fertility patterns and signs, opening the possibility to a slight change in Natural Family Planning's effectiveness. This is why the League created its special postpartum class.

The League also has created *The Art of Breastfeeding Diary*, a helpful aid for women who want to understand how breastfeeding impacts their return to fertility.

Contact the Couple to Couple League at www.ccli.org to obtain a copy.

Couples hoping to space pregnancies further apart than what is afforded them by lactation need to understand that the transition state can be complex, unique, and sometimes confusing. Once fertility signs reappear, patterns may shift depending upon breastfeeding frequency and intensity, which change throughout breastfeeding. Look beyond predictors and chart all fertility observations. Analyze changes in breastfeeding frequency including any change in night feedings, illnesses that affect breastfeeding, significant weight loss or addition of strenuous exercise, and introduction of complementary foods. All of these clues help identify and pinpoint your current phase of fertility, whether bleeding is menses or a "warning period," and whether the cycle has the potential to support a new pregnancy.

If your observations indicate you may be fertile yet you and your husband have discerned a need to postpone pregnancy, responsible parenthood suggests practicing abstinence during the fertile phase. And, expect the phases of fertility to be longer than they had been prior to pregnancy. Breastfeeding is a transition state. It is not unusual to experience slightly different fertility cycles throughout this transition due to the variables introduced by breastfeeding. It will not be until you reach your post-weaning cycles that you will feel you have returned to "regular" fertility.

The complexity and rigor of managing your fertility through the transition state can be eased by education, prayer and connecting with those who share your values, and parenting and marital goals. If you are unfamiliar with the rules of Natural Family Planning, the Couple to Couple League offers classes in the Sympto-Thermal Method across the country. Contact your local CCL chapter, or look online at http://www.ccli.org for a class near you, or purchase CCL's *Home Study Course*.

How breastfeeding and Natural Family Planning connect

As you and your husband prepare to resume a marital sexual relationship after childbirth, you both will want to understand how breastfeeding affects fertility, sexuality, child spacing, and responsible parenthood.

Some women may experience decreased libido while breastfeeding.

Many factors can contribute to this decline, including but not limited to fatigue, postpartum discomfort, decreased estrogen production, fear of pregnancy, and the demands of caring for a baby. Increasing libido, when accompanied by other fertility signs, can be one more clue to fertility's return.

Fear of pregnancy should not preclude couples from choosing to breastfeed their babies. Couples with serious reason to postpone pregnancy can effectively apply Natural Family Planning while breastfeeding. The abstinence required during fertile phases, while at times significant during the transition state, can continue to unify couples as they grow in how they express their love for each other in non-sexual ways, as they work through their frustrations, and as they communicate their hopes and dreams for the family that now includes a new baby. The art of Natural Family Planning fully supports the art of breastfeeding, and vice versa.

By now, you have learned a great deal about the art of breastfeeding and much, much more. You have learned that breastfeeding can provide you a natural period of infertility — a period of rest and healing — while also allowing you the opportunity to nurture your baby and provide him with the best available nutrition. You have also learned how your commitment to breastfeeding can impact your fertility and what signals to expect your body to send you as fertility resumes. The more you know about how your reproductive system responds to breastfeeding, the more confidently you will practice the art of breastfeeding in conjunction with the art of Natural Family Planning®. In the realm of fertility awareness, knowledge allows you to make better choices for yourself, for your baby, and for your marriage. You're becoming a master in the art of breastfeeding!

CHAPTER 8

Nutrition, Exercise and Weight Loss

The Couple to Couple League encourages exclusive breastfeeding for babies until age six months and continued breastfeeding until baby-led weaning occurs. This natural baby-led weaning process may occur anywhere between twelve months and thirty-six months or even later. We know that breastfeeding is strongly supported by the American College of Obstetrics and Gynecology, the American Academy of Family Physicians, the Academy of Breastfeeding Medicine, the World Heath Organization, the United Nations' Children's Fund, the La Leche League, and the American Academy of Pediatrics. Most agree there should be no upper limit to the duration of breastfeeding and there's no evidence of psychological or developmental harm from breastfeeding into a child's third year of life or longer.

We learned in chapter three about the various factors that can impact your breastfeeding success. One thing women do not often consider is the direct and indirect role nutrition plays in health, including before and during pregnancy, during lactation, and with regard to their fertility. All new mothers are encouraged to breastfeed, even if this means making dietary adjustments necessary to sustain maternal and infant health. Just as women choose to breastfeed for the big eight benefits (nutrition, psychological, health, environmental, economic, immunological, developmental, social), if you eat well, get adequate rest, and exercise during lactation those same benefits will be yours to enjoy.

While this book does not specifically address issues surrounding pregnancy, it is widely accepted that nutritional habits, which can impact lactation, are often formed during pregnancy. Marilyn Shannon, nutritionist and author of *Fertility, Cycles & Nutrition*, states that the vast majority of a person's well-being is directly affected through diet, the amount of rest they receive, and their level of exercise. When these three factors are in balance, expect to enjoy relatively good health. Similarly, feeling good during lactation merely hinges on achieving a good balance of diet, exercise, and rest. There are no extremes required. One should not shift to a restrictive diet or eat like there's no tomorrow or believe they need to "eat for two." One needn't take on excessive training such as might be required for a triathlon, but neither should one stop simple exercise like walking, riding a bicycle, or swimming. Adequate rest, especially immediately postpartum, may be harder to come by, but napping can be a good way to supplement rest missed during the night. The key is finding and maintaining balance.

Defining sound nutrition

We explained in chapter four that one barrier to breastfeeding is the misperception that a breastfeeding woman's diet needs to be severely restricted, with some favorite foods avoided. High quality milk production does not require special foods nor restrictive diets; it requires a balance of nutritious foods and avoidance of alcohol, tobacco, or anything that causes upset in either mother or baby. How well a woman eats during lactation affects her own health more than it will affect her ability to produce milk.

There are several schools of thought on what, exactly, constitutes healthy eating. One can look to the U.S. Department of Agriculture's "My Pyramid" for guidance (http://www.mypyramid.gov/). Guidelines have also been issued by the Harvard School for Public Health (http://www.hsph.harvard.edu/nutritionsource/) and the University of Michigan (http://www.med.umich.edu/umim/clinical/pyramid/index.htm). People with ethnic preferences can turn to the Asian Diet Pyramid, the Latin American Diet Pyramid, or the Mediterranean Diet Pyramid. A simple internet search will lead you to these guidelines and others. A vegetarian food pyramid is also available. All of these guidelines make unique distinctions for various food groups. Your preferences will determine which guidelines are most appropriate for you and your family. (Caution: vegan diets are inappropriate for lactation as they may result in unbalanced input of proteins, vitamins, minerals, and calories.)

The basic tenet to healthy eating is to limit discretionary (empty) calories, trans fats, and sugar. Healthy diets include: assorted fruits; vegetables; carbohydrates; meats and beans; the milk, yogurt and cheese group; and healthy fats. Diets that combine red meat, fish, poultry, beans, and nuts for protein offer numerous health benefits. Fruit and fruit juice are not interchangeable; "fruit juice" is not a suitable replacement for fresh fruit.

Fresh, unprocessed foods are considered the top of the food hierarchy with respect to nutrition, taste, and satisfaction. Frozen is better than canned fruits and vegetables. Fruits and vegetables canned in heavy syrups are not as good as those canned in natural juices. Steaming vegetables is better than boiling them since precious nutrients can get lost in the water used for boiling. Of course, eating fruits and vegetables

---

SOME FOODS CAN CAUSE ALLERGIC REACTIONS IN INFANTS

Not all foods commonly believed to cause upset will become problematic for your baby. Don't avoid a favorite food unless you consistently recognize one of these symptoms of distress in baby:[1]

A stuffy, itchy or drippy nose	Irritation in the diaper area
Irritation or redness of the eyes, tearing, or dark circles under the eyes	Fretful sleep
	Spitting up or vomiting
Pulling off the breast	Diarrhea, gas or green stool
Poor weight gain	Wheezing or coughing
Crying or colicky behavior	Asthma
Scaly or oily rashes	Chronic ear infections
Eczema	

These signs normally appear within hours of mother consuming an offending food.

A woman who has a food allergy or intolerance shouldn't worry about providing her baby with adequate nutrition if she continues to avoid problem foods while breastfeeding. How well a mother eats during lactation has less effect on her ability to make milk than on her own well being.[2]

[1] Lauwers, Judith, Swisher, Anna; *Counseling the Nursing Mother*, (Jones and Bartlett, 2005) 265

[2] Riordan, *Breastfeeding and Human Lactation*, 453.

raw is better than steaming because handling, cooking, or preserving foods alters the quality.

Whole grains are better than enriched or re-fortified grains, which turn to sugar quickly in digestion. Whole grains slow digestion, keeping blood sugar and insulin levels from rising too rapidly, an added benefit to keep hunger at bay. Whole grain food choices include: oatmeal, whole wheat bread, some crackers, pasta, tortillas, cornmeal, popcorn, bulgur, rye, quinoa, sorghum, amaranth, millet, and brown or wild rice. Whole grains are more expensive to buy and take longer to cook, consequently, one does not often encounter whole grains when eating at restaurants.

Organic foods are a popular choice as they do not contain pesticides or hormones; organics are increasingly becoming available in mainstream grocery stores. A good source for fresh, natural and organically-produced foods is your local farmer's market.

Food labels reveal good information about nutrition, but still fall short on full-disclosure. The main ingredient will be listed first on the label with subsequent ingredients listed in the order they appear by volume or weight. Additives are also listed. Some labels indicate whether the food item was grown or prepared as kosher, organic, and free of other common allergens such as peanuts, wheat, casein, etc. Food labels list the percentage of USDA recommended daily allowances met by the ingredients.

Foods labeled "low in fat" are often high in added sugar or sodium, which is not a good thing. Labels do not necessarily differentiate naturally occurring fats or sugars from added fats or sugars, making it difficult to gauge whether a processed product is "truly" a good choice.

Regardless of whether produce is organic or non-organic, all fruits and vegetables should be thoroughly washed before consuming. Chemical additives such as food coloring, fungicides, or waxes added at the grocery story to enhance the appearance of freshness can alter an item's taste and nutritional quality.

Lactating women should not skip meals or consume most of their day's calories at the last meal of the day. Instead, spread calorie intake evenly throughout the day to avoid hunger, which can lead to poor food choices. The human body performs at peak efficiency and endurance when calories are consumed evenly throughout the day.

Do not place undue stress on yourself by forcing yourself to adhere to some strict diet of "correct" foods. If you find that your everyday eating habits sustain you and give you adequate energy, there will be little need to alter your diet. Furthermore, the extra energy required by lactation is quite low — less than five hundred extra calories per day. The old adage about "eating for two" is unwise. Pregnancy and breastfeeding should not become an excuse for excessive eating or giving into cravings that may drive up calorie intake without providing essential nutrients. Good eating habits are learned early and will impact the overall health of your baby and your family, perhaps for generations. Even if you are new to the idea of eating healthy, take heart. Researchers at Cornell University in Ithaca, New York, found that women who understand how important good nutrition is to their lives and how it can impact their babies' outcomes can, and did, make positive changes in their food choices as they transitioned into motherhood.

A slight increase in protein intake is important during lactation. Non-lactating women require 59 grams of pure protein per day. Sixty grams per day is recommended during pregnancy and 65 grams per day is recommended during early lactation (up to baby's sixth month). After six months postpartum, protein intake can be reduced to 62 grams per day.[2] The protein content found in red meat is roughly seven grams per ounce. Other protein sources include dairy, vegetables, legumes and nuts. When choosing meat or poultry as a protein source, choose lean cuts, trim fat and skin, and avoid organ meats and highly processed meats such as bacon, sausages, and cold cuts.

Pregnant and lactating women need to be concerned with their intake of many varieties of fish. Dioxin, PCBs and mercury are commonly found in the environment and have shown up in many species of wild-caught fish. Pregnant women, young children and lactating mothers should exercise caution when choosing fish, including shellfish. Farm raised fish consumed in moderation, or wild-caught Alaskan Sockeye salmon, is an acceptable choice for pregnant and lactating women interested in consuming fish.[3]

Fats provide humans with the most concentrated source of energy available. Fats also act as the carriers for various fat soluble vitamins such as A, D, E, and K. Fats also prolong digestion by slowing down the stomach emptying time — tiding us over until our next meal. So, fats are important to our diet, but only as long as we choose good fats.

Fats are either classified as saturated or unsaturated. Saturated fats are primarily derived from animal sources such as meats, milk, and eggs. Unsaturated fats sources are vegetables, nuts, and seeds. A good diet contains more unsaturated fats than saturated fats; unsaturated fats decrease the risk of disease, thus they are considered *good* fats. The *bad* fats are those that tend to increase the risk of certain diseases and include both saturated and trans fats. Trans fats and saturated fats raise "bad" cholesterol levels increasing our risk of coronary heart disease. Trans fats can be found in most processed foods, including cakes, cookies, crackers, pies, bread, margarines, fried potatoes, and snack foods. Shortening and salad dressings also may contain trans fats.

Saturated fats are fats that exist naturally in animal products such as meat, dairy, eggs, and seafood. Some plant foods are also high in saturated fats, including coconut oils, palm oils, and palm kernel oils. The U.S. Food and Drug Administration recommends that consumers choose foods low in saturated fats and cholesterol; it also recommends that consumers check out food supplemental facts panels on products before purchasing. A 5 percent or lower rating for total fat, as reported on the daily value supplemental facts panel, is considered to be low or good; a total fat rating of 20 percent or higher means the item has too much bad cholesterol or saturated fat and should be avoided. The FDA also states: saturated fats are the "main dietary culprit that raises bad cholesterol (LDL) but trans fats and dietary cholesterol also contribute significantly."

The key to consuming fats is to substitute good fats for bad fats whenever possible. A low-fat diet that eliminates the *good* fats along with the *bad* fats is not necessarily healthy. A *very* low-fat diet is not normally appropriate during pregnancy or lactation.

Vitamins are needed for the body to convert fats and carbohydrates into energy. They also help form bone and tissue. Vitamin supplements may be acceptable for lactating women as long as they are not used to replace foods naturally high in vitamins and minerals. Look for multi-vitamin and multi-mineral supplements that meet requirements of the

United States Pharmacopeia, the organization that sets standards for drugs and supplements. Lactating mothers are cautioned to steer clear of drugs or vitamin supplements (including vitamin B6 exceeding 4 mg/day) that suppress milk production.[4]

A developing infant requires a great deal of calcium with mother being the source. This leads to a bone mineral loss in mother that is only temporary. Research reveals that calcium levels will return to pre-pregnancy levels, or higher, once lactation ceases.[5] A woman who is concerned about her calcium intake during lactation is advised to use calcium carbonate, especially if she is under age twenty-five and is still building her own calcium stores. Lactating women should get 1,200 milligrams of calcium per day. Women who are lactose intolerant may be heartened to learn that milk consumption is in no way related to milk production.

Lactational amenorrhea can offset a mother's need for additional iron, therefore iron supplements are rarely required during lactation.

Iodine is important for lactating women and 150 micro-grams per day is the recommended dose. Iodine is found in kelp, iodized salt, and seafood.

Water is the most important nutrient in and for the body, and is involved in every bodily function. Normally, women find lactation will increase thirst. Lactating mothers are advised to drink at least eight cups of water per day, more when perspiring heavily. Lactating women should drink enough water to quench thirst and should stay alert to signs of dehydration — dry skin, dry eyes, and reduced urine output. Water loss through perspiration and excretion can equal two quarts per day.

While dehydration can lead to reduced milk volume, lactating women are also cautioned to avoid excessive water consumption as studies have shown it can lead to decreased weight gain in infants and a higher risk of mother experiencing dangerous water toxicity. There is no correlation between increasing water intake and increased milk volume.

For some mothers, the first sign of dehydration is constipation. For others, adequate hydration can be gauged by urine color; under normal circumstances, urine should be clear to light yellow. Dark urine is a hint that hydration has been compromised; intake of even just two cups per day less than what is recommended causes a mild degree of dehydration. A goal for water consumption is to eliminate thirst, maintain bodily fluid stores, and avoid dehydration. Even fruit is a good source for chemically pure water.

The purpose of pursuing sound nutrition while breastfeeding is simple: any substance that goes into your body will find its way into breast milk and, ultimately, into your baby. If you eat properly, baby will prosper; if you eat poorly, both of you could suffer.

Environmental pollutants

There are other substances that can affect breast milk that are not directly ingested, such as environmental chemicals or pollutants. News reports about toxins appearing in breast milk have recently emerged, concerning many. It is true that industrial toxins, such as dioxins, PCBs, mercury, phthalates, pesticides, flame retardants, and others, pass through the placenta and into a fetus during pregnancy and also appear in breast milk of exposed mothers. A statement by the National Resource Defense Council indicates a mother's exposure to environmental toxins is not cause to stop breastfeeding. As you learned in chapter two, the protective effect of breastfeeding is monumental and can help limit the damage caused by fetal exposure.[6]

Contaminants exist in artificial formulas (and in commercial infant foods), yet manufactured formula lacks the immunological benefits of sterile breast milk.

It is prudent, however, to reduce your exposure to chemical contaminants by:

> Not smoking and avoiding second-hand smoke.

> Avoid eating fish species known to be high in mercury.

> Avoid contaminants common to the home, such as pesticides, fertilizers, some cleaning products, paints, solvents, stripping solutions, nail polish, perfume, gasoline fumes, and solvent-based glues.

> Choose organic products.

> Wash produce thoroughly before consuming.

Shedding those pregnancy pounds

Maintaining weight is a matter of simple math: when the intake of calories equals energy expended, weight remains steady. If your goal is weight loss, you must alter the equation; either decrease your input (eat less) or increase expended energy (exercise more). A combination of the two is the most effective way to lose weight *and* maintain weight loss. Your continued good health hinges on achieving a proper balance between good diet and exercise.

During the first two weeks after delivery, your thoughts should not fall on your diet. It is critical to establish milk supply immediately post-partum; your efforts here will go a long way toward helping you achieve your pre-pregnancy weight as long as you do not over-eat. Consuming 1,800 calories per day is the absolute minimum for mothers who are exclusively breastfeeding. Lactating women can consume 2,220 calories per day and still lose weight. It is not until consumption reaches roughly 2,600 calories per day when weight loss stops. The ideal rate of postpartum weight loss is between one and two pounds per month.

Lactating women should not use liquid diet shakes or other diet medications; their additives and active ingredients will find their way into breast milk.

One of the biggest challenges to healthy eating and achieving weight loss after giving birth is pulling together nutritious meals when you are tired and stressed trying to meet the demands of a new baby and grow-ing family. Resist the urge to pull frozen dinners from the freezer or run to fast food restaurants; these meals are expensive, not as nutritious as home-cooked meals, and can be heavily laden with fat, sugar, and so-dium. It may be helpful to plan meals a week out to avoid last-minute scrambling. See Appendix D for other helpful suggestions on how to eat healthy and save money.

Moderate exercise will not adversely affect lactation. The key word here is moderate. Slow, steady weight loss through sound nutrition and moderate exercise should be your goal; lactation is no time to train for a marathon.

When exercising, the following tips may be helpful: It is a good idea to pump before exercising, for two reasons. First, pumping will reduce some of the pressure full breasts can place on you during motion. Secondly, exercise builds lactic acid, which can leach into breast milk, changing its pH and taste. If, after exercising, you notice baby refusing to feed or pulling away from the breast, he may be reacting to this bitter lactic acid in the milk. Breast milk normally tastes sweet so this exercise-induced change in taste may startle him. If lactic acid is present in your breast milk, pump a small amount from each breast, less than an eighth of a cup, and discard it; lactic acid is more likely to be present only in the early milk. If baby refuses to breastfeed after exercise, the milk you pumped earlier can be used for a post-exercise feeding.

Another thing baby could react to after exercise is the salty taste of your perspiration. Always shower after exercise and before attempting to breastfeed. Also, be sure to wear an extremely supportive, well fitting bra to help reduce any friction from movement.

In conclusion, you can see it does not take an exceptional diet to practice the art of breastfeeding but it may require making some minor adjustments to your pre-pregnancy eating and drinking habits. Usually, these adjustments benefit both mother and baby.

If you are concerned about getting back into shape after childbirth, be patient. Moderation in exercise and eating are keys to enjoying a healthy lifestyle, even when not lactating, and these two also facilitate weight loss. Remember the axiom: calorie intake must be lower than energy expended for weight loss to occur. Eating well nutritionally, exercising, and getting adequate rest will help you get back into shape fastest.

Conclusion

Breastfeeding is a very unique human experience because it welcomes mothers into the process of learning about their babies so that they may nourish and nurture them. Breastfeeding is an art; women who successfully practice it convey nourishment and love along with all the other proven benefits. These women are artisans — they've mastered the art of breastfeeding. Now you can, too.

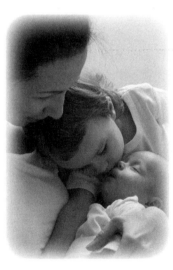

As a mother who breastfeeds, you interact with your baby in a truly unique way. Your breast milk is a "living substance" that maximizes his growth, health, and nutrition while also providing emotional reassurance through your gaze, your voice, your touch. Your interaction increases your baby's cognitive capacity while he receives the sterile, perfect nutrition designed uniquely for him. If your world included only the two of you, breastfeeding until baby-led weaning would be simple.

But the two of you do not exist in a vacuum. Your decision to breastfeed and your determination to continue will impact you, your husband, other children in the family, and society — in ways you may not have expected. Ideally, the decision to breastfeed is one you will make together with your husband. If this is your first baby, the choice to breastfeed can be an early example of how both parents need to be in sync on important child-rearing decisions.

Another reason you'll want the full support of your husband is that research has shown he can be your best ally when breastfeeding challenges emerge. This book offers ample evidence of why breastfeeding can be considered a worthwhile activity, one that brings joy, yet also involves some sacrifice.

The pattern of the whole of breastfeeding, i.e., the eight benefits reaped by baby, mother, father, and society, is truly the sum of each of its parts. In other words, each breastfeeding benefit, whether it is healthful, nutritional, immunologic, psychological, developmental, social, environmental, or economic, makes breastfeeding best for baby, mother, father and society. Yet one cannot master the whole of breastfeeding — the art of breastfeeding — by focusing on only one or two of its parts, or benefits. The art of breastfeeding is achieved when one appreciates the whole of the parts, all the benefits combined.

The degree to which breastfeeding could be considered "hard work" will depend on your commitment to providing your baby with his best possible outcome and the degree of support your commitment receives from others. The "hardest" part of breastfeeding is often just getting others to acknowledge that breastfeeding is "best" for babies, moms, dads, families, and society. If you encounter detractors, enlist your husband's help as you reexamine the facts offered here and together, share this information with others.

Furthermore, be patient with yourself as you practice the art of breastfeeding and seek out a certified lactation consultant as soon as you encounter those tough-to-overcome difficulties that can threaten your success. Because breastfeeding's benefits are so crucial to baby's development, you will want to build a support network to help you get through the difficult periods when your commitment to continued breastfeeding may wane. And remember not to buy into the claims made by manufacturers, which promote infant formula to be "most like mother's milk." The evidence is clear; breast milk is best for baby! Furthermore, the days you spend breastfeeding your baby will likely count among the most rewarding and fulfilling days of your life. In that regard, breastfeeding is best for mothers too!

Today's mother is smart, educated, and she enjoys more freedom than any generation that came before her. It is the sophistication of today's women which accounts for breastfeeding's growth in popularity in recent years in the United States, though breastfeeding rates are still lower than in other countries, especially for older babies. Mothers are waking up to the fact that the pace of American society is leading women and their children into dangerous territory, with increases seen in childhood diabetes and childhood obesity rates. Breastfeeding is a way for women and their babies to slow down and reverse this disturbing trend.

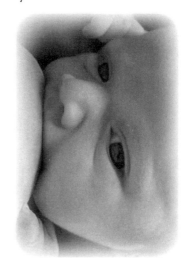

When a woman makes breastfeeding a priority, she is committing herself to insuring a better future for her baby, with added benefits for her, her husband, their family, and all of society. Women who choose to breastfeed reorder their priorities away from the empty promises made by the prevailing culture and place the good of their families ahead of pursuits that often involve self. All women who give birth will come to realize that motherhood brings with it choices that involve sacrifice. It is the women who commit to continued breastfeeding who will become well-versed in the act of sacrifice.

In this vein, breastfeeding is the fulfillment of God's design for women. For it is through sacrifice that we can experience the fullness of God's love for us and it is the giving of self through breastfeeding that a woman can express her undying love for her baby. Furthermore, it is through a baby's complete dependence on his mother and her response to his dependence, through breastfeeding, that mother and child reinforce each other's dignity.

For family life to flourish, a commitment by all involved is required. It is the same with the art of breastfeeding. If you wish to be successful learning and practicing the art of breastfeeding, you must commit yourself to the process the same way an artist commits to his art. Love the process. Love your baby. Love yourself. And may God bless you.

Endnotes

Chapter 2 endnotes

[1] Lawrence, Ruth, *Tribute to Paul Gyorgy* (Breastfeeding Medicine 2006): 1:1

[2] American Academy of Pediatrics, *Breastfeeding and the Use of Human Milk* (Pediatrics 1997) 100:6, 1035-1039, http://aappolicy.aapublications.org/cgi/content/full/pediatrics;100/6/1035

[3] Lawrence, Ruth; Lawrence, Robert, *Breastfeeding: A Guide for the Medical Professional* (Elsevier Mosby 2005) 1026-27

[4] Ibid. 1027

[5] Lauwers, Judith; Swisher, Anna, *Counseling the Nursing Mother* (Jones and Bartlett, 2005): 139

[6] Riordon, Jan, *Breastfeeding and Human Lactation* (Jones and Bartlett 2005): 527

[7] Lauwers, Judith; Swisher, Anna, *Counseling the Nursing Mother* (Jones and Bartlett, 2005): 162

[8] Akobeng, A.K.; Ramanan; A.V., Buchan, I; Heller, R.F.; *Effect of Breastfeeding on Risk of Celiac Disease: a Systematic Review and Meta-analysis of Observational Studies*, (Archives of Childhood Diseases 2006) 91;39-43

[9] Palmer, Brian; *The Influence of Breastfeeding on the Development of the Oral Cavity: A commentary*, (Journal of Human Lactation, 1998)

[10] Lauwers, Judith; Swisher, Anna, *Counseling the Nursing Mother* (Jones and Bartlett, 2005): 116

[11] Newcomb, Polly, Et al., *Lactation and a Reduced risk of Pre-menopausal Breast Cancer*, (New England Journal of Medicine 1994): 330:81-87:2, 8

[12] Ibid: 330:81-87:2, 2-9

[13] AbuSabha, Rayanne and Greene, Geoffrey, *Body Weight, Body Composition, and Energy Intake Changes in Breastfeeding Mothers*, (Journal of Human Lactation 1998): 119

[14] Lauwers, Judith; Swisher, Anna, *Counseling the Nursing Mother* (Jones and Bartlett, 2005): 135

[15] Riordan, Jan, *Breastfeeding and Human Lactation,* (Jones and Bartlett 2005): 100

[16] Uauy, Ricardo; Peirano, Patricio, *Breast is Best: Human Milk is the Optimal Food for Brain Development,* (American Journal of Clinical Nutrition, 1999): 70:433-434

[17] Anderson, James; Johnstone, Bryan, and Remley, Daniel, *Breastfeeding and Cognitive Development: A Meta-Analysis,* (The American Journal of Clinical Nutrition 1990) 70:525-35

[18] Mennella, Julia, *Mother's Milk: A Medium for Early Flavor Experiences,* (Journal for Human Lactation 1995): 11:1, 35-45

[19] American Heart Association, Et al., *Dietary Recommendations for Children and Adolescents: A Guide for Practitioners,* (Pediatrics 2007) 117:544-559

[20] Gribble, Karleen, *Mental Health, Attachment and Breastfeeding: Implications for Adopted Children and their Mothers,* (International Breastfeeding Journal 2006) 1:5, 2

[21] Weimer, Jon, *The Economic Benefits of Breastfeeding,* (Economic Research Service/USDA 2001): 3

Chapter 3 endnotes

1 Moran, Victoria, et al; *Breastfeeding Support for Adolescent Mothers: Similarities and Differences in the Approach of Midwives and Qualified Breastfeeding Supporters* (International Breastfeeding Journal, 2006) 1:23

2 Walker, Marcia, *Breastfeeding Management for the Clinician* (Jones and Bartlett 2006): 154

3 Smith, Linda, *ABC Protocol for Solving Breastfeeding Problems* (1993, 2000) http://www.bflrc.com/ and International Lactation Consultant Association, *Evidence Based Guidelines for Breastfeeding Management During the First Fourteen Days,* (2005) http://www.ilca.org/research.html

4 Ibid., 151

5 Ibid., 150-151

6 Smith, *ABC Protocol for Solving Breastfeeding Problems*

7 Ibid., 303

8 Lauwers, Judith, Swisher, Anna, *Counseling the Nursing Mother* (Jones and Bartlett, 2005): 320

9 Ibid: 320

10 Ibid: 320

11 Smith, *ABC Protocol for Solving Breastfeeding Problems*

12 Ibid

13 Radford, B.L. Philipp, *Baby-Friendly: Snappy Slogan or Standard of Care?,* (Archives of Diseases in Childhood; Fetal and Neonatal Edition 2006): 91:F145-149

[14] Lauwers, Judith, Swisher, Anna, *Counseling the Nursing Mother* (Jones and Bartlett, 2005): 264

Chapter 4 endnotes

[1] Thomas, Karen and Burr, *Robert, Preterm Infant Temperature Circadian Rhythm: Possible Effect of Parental Cosleeping*, (Biological Research for Nursing 2002) 3:3, 150-159

[2] Ibid., 151

[3] Heinig, Jane, *Bed Sharing and Infant Mortality: Guilt by Association?* (Journal of Human Lactation 2000) 16:3 190

[4] Weimer, Stephen, Et al, *Prevalence, Predictors, and Attitudes Toward Cosleeping in an Urban Pediatric Center* (Clinical Pediatrics 2002)41:436

[5] McKenna, James, *Sleeping with your Baby*, (Platypus Media 2007): 54-55

[6] American Association of Pediatrics, http://aappolicy.aappublications.org/cgi/content/full/pediatrics%3b105/3/650

[7] McKenna, *Sleeping with your Baby*, 73

[8] Weimer, *Prevalence, Predictors, and Attitudes Toward Cosleeping in an Urban Pediatric Center*, 435

[9] American Association of Pediatrics, *Changing Concepts of Sudden Infant Death Syndrome: Implications for Infant Sleeping Environment and Sleep Position*, (Pediatrics 2000) 105:3, 650-656

[10] Ibid. 650

Chapter 5 endnotes

[1] Nommsen-Rivers, Laurie, *Cosmetic Breast Surgery: Is Breastfeeding at Risk?* (*Journal of Human Lactation* 2003) 19:1

[2] Lawrence, Ruth, *Breastfeeding: A Guide for the Medical Profession*, (Elsevier 2005): 357

[3] Riordan, *Breastfeeding and Human Lactation*, 636

Chapter 6 endnotes

[1] Lauwers, Judith and Swisher, Anna, *Counseling the Nursing Mother* (Jones and Bartlett 2005): 340

[2] American Heart Association, *Dietary Recommendations for Children and Adolescents: A Guide for Practitioners*, 550

[3] Kendall-Tackett, Kathleen, and Sugarman, Muriel, *The Social Consequences of Long-term Breastfeeding*, (Journal of Human Lactation 1995) 11:3, 179

[4] Stein, Martin, Boies, Eyla, and Snyder, David, *Parental Concerns about*

Extended Breastfeeding in a Toddler, (Pediatrics 2004): 114:1506-1509

5 Lauwers, *Counseling the Nursing Mother*, 355

6 Ibid., 340

Chapter 7 endnotes

1 Van Look, P., and von Hertzen, H., *World Health Organization Multinational Study of Breastfeeding and Lactational Amenorrhea*, (Elsevier 1998): 70:3, 465

2 Taylor, H.W., et al, *Continuously Recorded Suckling Behavior and its Effect on Lactational Amenorrhea*, (Journal of Biosocial Science 1999) 31:289-310

3 Ibid., 289-310

4 Lawrence, Ruth, *Breastfeeding: A Guide for the Medical Profession*, (Elsevier 2005): 739

5 Ibid., 747

6 Ibid., 742

7 *Breastfeeding: Maternal and Infant Aspects* (ACOG Educational Bulletin, July 2000): No. 258

8 Liebert, Mary Ann, *ABM Clinical Protocol #13, Contraception During Breast-feeding*, (Breastfeeding Medicine 2006) 1:1, 49

Chapter 8 endnotes

1 *Breastfeeding and the Use of Human Milk*, (AAP Policy, Dec. 1, 1997) 1-40

2 Ibid., 448

3 http://www.deliciousorganics.com/Controversies/foodcontroversies.htm

4 Lauwers, *Counseling the Nursing Mother*, 135

5 Lawrence, *Breastfeeding, A Guide for the Medical Profession*, 240

6 Natural Resources Defense Council, *Toward Healthy Environments for Children*, http://www.nrdc.org

Appendix A

Online Sources for Information on Pregnancy, Childbirth, Breastfeeding and Natural Family Planning

The Couple to Couple League
(800) 745-8252
www.ccli.org

Academy of Breastfeeding Medicine*
http://www.bfmed.org/

Baby Friendly, USA*
http://www.babyfriendlyusa.org/

Breastfeeding and Human Lactation Study Center*
http://usbreastfeeding.org/breastfeeding/compend-bhlsc.htm

International Childbirth Education Association*
http://www.icea.org/

International Lactation Consultant Association*
http://www.ilca.org

*The Couple to Couple League does not endorse these organizations; it merely offers them as a resource for breastfeeding information and support.

La Leche League*
http://www.llli.org/

Natural Childbirth Association*
http://www.birthingnaturally.net/

One More Soul
http://www.omsoul.com/

Pope Paul VI Institute
http://www.popepaulvi.com/

Wellstart International*
http://www.wellstart.org/resources.html

World Alliance for Breastfeeding Action*
http://www.waba.org.my/

Appendix B

Baby-Friendly Hospitals as of 2007

CALIFORNIA

Barstow Community Hospital, Barstow
Community Hospital of San Bernardino
Community Hospital of the Monterey Peninsula, Monterey
Corona Regional Medical Center, Corona
Glendale Memorial Hospital and Health Center, Glendale
Goleta Valley Cottage Hospital, Santa Barbara
Inland Midwife Services - The Birth Center, Redlands
Kaiser Permanente Medical Center, Hayward
Kaiser Permanente Riverside Medical Center, Riverside
Mountains Community Hospital, Lake Arrowhead
Providence Holy Cross Medical Center, Mission Hills
Robert E. Bush Naval Hospital, Twenty-nine Palms
Scripps Memorial Hospital Encinitas
San Francisco General Hospital, San Francisco
UCSD Medical Center, San Diego
Ventura County Medical Center, Ventura
Weed Army Community Hospital, Fort Irwin
Women's Health & Birth Center, Santa Rosa

COLORADO

Exempla Good Samaritan Medical Center, Lafayette

CONNECTICUT

Hartford Hospital, Hartford
Middlesex Hospital, Middletown

FLORIDA
Cape Canaveral Hospital, Cocoa Beach
Morton Plant Hospital, Clearwater

HAWAII
Kaiser Permanente Medical Center, Honolulu

IDAHO
Kootenai Medical Center, Coeur d'Alene

INDIANA
Community Hospital Anderson
Methodist Hospital, Indianapolis

ILLINOIS
St. John's Hospital, Springfield
Pekin Hospital, Pekin

KENTUCKY
St. Elizabeth Medical Center, Edgewood

MAINE
Central Maine Medical Center, Lewiston
Maine General Medical Center, Augusta & Waterville
Miles Memorial Hospital, Damariscotta

MASSACHUSETTS
Boston Medical Center, Boston

MONTANA
Community Hospital of Anaconda

NEBRASKA
Methodist Hospital, Omaha

NEW HAMPSHIRE
Alice Peck Day Memorial Hospital, Lebanon
St. Joseph Hospital, Nashua

NEW YORK

Rochester General Hospital, Rochester

OHIO

Mercy Hospital Anderson, Cincinnati
Mercy Hospital Fairfield

OREGON

Kaiser Sunnyside Medical Center, Clackamas
Peace Health Nurse Midwifery Birth Center, Eugene
Providence Medford Medical Center, Medford
Three Rivers Community Hospital, Grants Pass

PENNSYLVANIA

Reading Birth & Women's Center, Reading

RHODE ISLAND

Newport Hospital, Newport
South County Hospital, Wakefield

TENNESSEE

Lisa Ross Birth & Women's Center, Knoxville
Women's Wellness & Maternity Center, Madisonville

VERMONT

Northeastern Vermont Regional Hospital, St. Johnsbury

WASHINGTON

Evergreen Hospital Medical Center, Kirkland
Okanogan-Douglas District Hospital, Brewster
St. Mary Medical Center, Walla Walla
Tacoma General Hospital, Tacoma

WISCONSIN

Aurora Lakeland Medical Center, Elkhorn
Elmbrook Memorial Hospital, Brookfield

Madison Birth Center, Middleton
Meriter Hospital, Madison
St. Francis Hospital, Milwaukee

GERMANY

US Army MEDDAC, Heidelberg

Source: http://www.babyfriendlyusa.org

Appendix C

Human donor milk provides most of the beneficial, species specific properties found in mother's milk, which makes it the ideal nutrition source for infants when a mother cannot provide her infant with her own milk through breastfeeding or pumping. (See the Hierarchy of Infant Feeding in chapter two.) Donor milk has proven to be a life saver for many infants whose mother's milk is unavailable.

Human Milk Banks

CALIFORNIA

Mothers' Milk Bank, San Jose
(408) 998-4550

COLORADO

Mothers' Milk Bank at Presbyterian St. Luke's Medical Center, Denver
(877) 458-5503

DELAWARE

Mothers' Milk Bank, Christiana Hospital, Newark
(302)733-3320

INDIANA

Indiana Mothers' Milk Bank, Inc., Methodist Medical Plaza II, Indianapolis
(317) 329-7146

IOWA

Mother's Milk Bank of Iowa, University of Iowa Hospitals and Clinics, Iowa City
(319)356-2652

MASSACHUSETTS

Mothers' Milk Bank of New England, Newtonville
(617) 964-6676

MICHIGAN

Bronson Mothers' Milk Bank, Kalamazoo
(269) 341-8849

NORTH CAROLINA

WakeMed Mothers' Milk Bank and Lactation Center, Raleigh
(919) 350-8599

OHIO

Mothers' Milk Bank of Ohio, Grant Medical Center, Columbus
(614) 544-0810

TEXAS

Mothers' Milk Bank at Austin
(512) 494-0800

Mothers' Milk Bank of North Texas, Ft. Worth
(817) 810-0071

BRITISH COLUMBIA, CANADA

BC Women's Milk Bank, C & W Lactation Services, Vancouver
604) 875-2282

Source: The Human Milk Banking Association of America, http://www.hmbana.org/

Home collection and storage of human milk

When breast milk is collected and stored for future home use, consideration needs to be given to preserve the safety and quality of this milk. How milk is collected and stored introduces the possibility for contamination, spoilage and reduced nutritional properties.

Always practice good hygiene when pumping and collecting milk.

Wash and sterilize equipment after each use and avoid cross contamination from other sources.

Store milk from each pumping session separately and label it with the time and date of collection. Breast milk not to be used within twenty-four hours should be frozen immediately after collected; do not refreeze once breast milk thaws. When thawing frozen milk, stir it to blend the fat that may cling to the side of the container. Also, never warm human milk in a microwave oven. Freshly expressed milk is preferred to frozen when baby is unable to breastfeed.

Equipment resources

Hand expression and hand-held pumps are suitable only for temporary relief of engorgement. Electric or hospital-grade breast pumps, while more expensive, are the best choice for women who expect pumping to have a significant role in feeding their babies. Electric pumps mimic baby's suck most efficiently, a critical feature for maintaining milk supply. Manufacturers that produce hospital-grade electric breast pumps include Medela, Avent, and Ameda (Hollister/Egnell).

One online source that offers side-by-side comparisons of various types of breast pumps can be found at: http://www.breastpumpsdirect.com/

The La Leche League also offers resources and information about pumping. http://www.llli.org/

Breast pumps can sometimes be rented. Check with your local hospital or the breastfeeding connection for information. Be cautious when renting or borrowing a breast pump. Be sure all parts are clean, sterile and in proper working condition. http://www.lactationconnection.com/breast_pump_rentals.aspx

Appendix D

Thirty-three ways to save money and eat healthier

Everyone wants to save money and keep grocery costs low. Here are some strategies to improve your nutrition and overall health while also saving money.

1. Produce in season is often less expensive. Buy asparagus in spring, zucchini in late summer, and pears in the fall.

2. Locate a farmer's market in your area. Local produce hasn't traveled long distances, so it is often in better condition and priced more affordably. Some areas offer community supported agriculture for families to subscribe to farm-fresh produce that can be delivered right to your doorstep.

3. Seek out pick-your-own farms for berries and other produce. This can also provide a good workout for the picker.

4. Grow your own herbs, vegetables and fruit in a backyard garden, patio, or sunny windowsill.

5. Buy only as much fresh produce as you will use within three or four days. Nutritional value decreases the longer produces sits, and throwing food away is wasteful. Overripe fruits like bananas and peaches can be used for baking.

6. Choose canned or frozen fruits and vegetables when fresh varieties are most expensive or unavailable. Remember to not add sugar and salt as frozen and canned goods contain these things. Always read food labels.

7. To prevent impulse buys, always prepare a grocery list when shopping.

8. Shop on a full stomach; hunger increases the chance you'll place unplanned purchases or unhealthy foods in your cart.

9. Use coupons only for products you were planning to buy anyway. Try to combine sale items with coupons for extra savings.

10. Try store brand or generic products; you may not find much difference between these and more expensive brand names.

11. Where bulk foods are available, choose to scoop your own grains, beans, cereals, nuts, etc. You will save money by buying only what you need.

12. Buy juices as frozen concentrate instead of ready-to-use in bottles or cartons. The nutritional content is the same. Choose only 100 percent fruit juices.

13. Buy plain brown rice or other whole grains and add your own herbs and spices instead of prepackaged blends.

14. Purchase plain, nonfat yogurt and add your own chopped apples, spices or vanilla. You'll get less sugar and it will cost less money.

15. Instead of buying a gallon of ice cream, buy popsicles or ice cream sandwiches. Try soy versions. Although individually wrapped packaged options cost more per unit, they will help you control portion sizes. If you eat less, you'll save money.

16. Decide which convenience foods are necessary. Would you rather slice mushrooms or tear your own lettuce leaves than buy prepackaged options? Or is the reduced preparation time worth the few extra dollars?

17. Consider joining a food co-op or membership store.

18. Make your own sandwiches so you can control portions.

Use less mayonnaise and heap on more veggies. Make sure to choose a fiber-rich whole grain bread.

19. Keep a bottle of water with you all day instead of buying sodas. Water has no calories, caffeine or sugar.

20. Bring your lunch to work. Stir fry or veggie pasta leftovers can be quickly heated in the microwave. There may even be time for a midday walk.

21. Rather than going to the vending machine, bring snacks from home: fresh-fruit salad, raisins or other dried fruits, unsalted nuts, raw veggies, baked tortilla chips, flavored rice cakes or crunchy whole grain cereal.

22. Instead of buying deli turkey by the pound, purchase a whole turkey breast, roast it in the oven, slice it into individual portions and freeze in zipper bags until needed. Turkey is perfect for quick sandwiches or salad toppings.

23. When you purchase meat, divide it into three-ounce servings, and place in freezer safe bags or containers. This helps control portion sizes and encourages you to use less meat in casseroles, stir fry and pasta sauces.

24. Always keep a few cans of beans on hand to use as a meat substitute in various dishes.

25. Cutting down on meat purchases leaves more money to buy a variety of vegetables, even out of season. Eating a variety of foods will make it easier to eat less meat.

26. When you are too tired or busy to cook a full meal, don't fall into the expensive trap of going out to a restaurant. Instead, make a veggie-filled sandwich or have soup and whole grain crackers.

27. Freeze leftovers rather than refrigerate them, unless you are sure you'll use them the next day.

28. Try making your own salad dressing with olive oil, flavored vinegar and your favorite seasonings.

29. Since baked goods freeze well, make muffins and quick breads in large quantities. Include whole grains, shredded vegetables and fresh or dried fruits.

30. Store-bought trail mix often contains excessive salt, sugar and saturated fat. Create you own trail mix with unsalted nuts, whole grain cereal, pretzels, and chopped dried fruits.

31. Remember that eating healthy now will save money on health costs in the future. Fill your plate with two-thirds vegetables, fruits, whole grains and beans and one-third, or less, animal foods.

32. When traveling, bring along a cooler with water, fruit, and healthy snacks.

33. Plan your menu for the entire week and plan purchases around weekly sales.

Source: University of California Cooperative Extension

Glossary

ALVEOLI: Small sacs in which milk is secreted and stored.

AMENORRHEA: An absence of menstrual bleeding. Lactational amenorrhea is the absence of menstrual bleeding due to breastfeeding.

AREOLA: Pigmented skin surrounding the nipple.

ATTACHMENT PARENTING: A parenting philosophy with multiple connotations and principles, which may or may not include breastfeeding.

BREAKTHROUGH BLEEDING: Flow of blood from the uterus not associated with ovulation.

BASAL BODY TEMPERATURE (BBT): Temperature of the body after a night's sleep that is unaffected by food, drink or activity. The Sympto-Thermal Method of natural family planning incorporates BBT into its method. BBT is measured orally at the same time each day.

BEHAVIORAL BREASTFEEDING ISSUES: Access to breast not sufficient to achieve proper outcomes for baby or maintain adequate milk supply.

BODY MASS INDEX: A formula that uses weight and height to estimate body fat and health risks.

BREASTFEEDING ISSUES: Problems encountered with breastfeeding that negatively impact baby, mother or both. There are two general categories of breastfeeding issues: behavioral and mechanical.

BUTTINSKY: One given to butting in; a troublesome meddler.

CASEIN: The principal protein in mammalian milk.

CIRCADIAN RHYTHM: Body temperature rises during the early morning hours and begins to fall in the evening. This normal rise and subsequent fall in body temperature is known as the circadian rhythm. Basal thermometers measure the temperature of the rested body unaffected by drink, food or activity at the same time within this circadian rhythm.

CLOSETED BREASTFEEDING: Refusing to breastfeed in public places or in the presence of others.

CLUSTER FEEDING: Frequently spaced breast feedings occurring back to back or in a shorter span of time than usually experienced. Cluster feedings are normal when they are the result of making up for lost feedings due to longer sleep periods, or when baby missed or delayed feedings for a variety of reasons (illness, busy mother, etc). Cluster feedings help make up lost calories due to delayed or missed feedings.

COITUS: Sexual intercourse.

COGNITIVE DEVELOPMENT: A complex process by which a baby's awareness and understanding (intellect) develops. Influenced by genetic and environmental factors that interact with each other. Breastfeeding and maternal bonding are influencers within these environmental factors.

COLOSTRUM: The fluid at the breast at the end of pregnancy and in the early postpartum period. Colostrum is thick and yellow reflecting high protein content; it is also high in vitamins A, E and K and minerals sodium and zinc.

COMPLEMENTARY FEEDING: Adding nutrition or food after a breastfeeding session when baby indicates continued hunger.

CONTINUED BREASTFEEDING: Breastfeeding that continues past the sixth month while offering complementary or supplementary feedings.

CO-SLEEPING: Has several implications, some of which may not be associated with breastfeeding. Co-sleeping may mean that mother and baby share a bed; it can also mean when mother and baby sleep in close proximity to each other but do not share the same bed.

DUCTS (LACTIFEROUS): The fifteen to twenty-four tubes in the breast, which collect milk from the smaller ductules and carry it to the nipple. Appearance is similar to stems on a branch of grapes, the alveoli being the grapes. The ducts open into nipple pores.

ECOLOGICAL BREASTFEEDING: A breastfeeding practice that calls for exclusive and extended breastfeeding with no bottles or pacifiers, schedules, or separation from baby including for naps and nighttime sleep.

EXCLUSIVE BREASTFEEDING: No other foods or liquids given to an infant prior to the sixth month.

FERTILITY CYCLE: A woman's reproductive cycle divided into three phases. *Phase I* relates to the infertile period of time from onset of menses until the first day of fertility. *Phase II* is the stage of fertility when pregnancy can be achieved. *Phase III* is another infertile period of time following ovulation and ending with the onset of menses.

FOLLICLE: Clusters of cells in the ovary capable of producing hormones; when properly stimulated, follicles release an ovum or egg.

FORE MILK: The milk obtained at the beginning of breastfeeding. Its higher water content keeps infants hydrated and supplies water-soluble vitamins and proteins.

HERBAL MEDICINES: A plant or plant part used for its therapeutic properties. Herbal medicine products are classified as dietary supplements; people take them to improve their health. They are sold as tablets, capsules, powders, teas, extracts and fresh or dried plants.

HIND MILK: Milk released later in a breastfeeding session (after 10 minutes). Hind milk is higher in fat, up to 6 percent or more; this is two to three times the fat concentration in fore milk.

HORMONES: Chemical signals produced by the body necessary to maintain cellular activity. Primary hormones affecting fertility cycles include: insulin, progesterone, estrogens, luteinizing hormone (LH), follicle stimulating hormone (FSH), prolactin and oxytocin.

IMMUNOLOGIC: Providing immunity to disease by stimulating antigens (a substance foreign to the body, often protein).

IMMUNOGLOBULIN: A group of five distinct antibodies (IgA, IgD, IgE, IgG, and IgM) in the blood and external secretions of the body that provide immunity.

INSUFFICIENT MILK SYNDROME: A mechanical issue complicating breastfeeding.

LACTATION: The secretion of human milk from the breast following pregnancy.

LACTOFERRIN: a human milk protein that "binds" or locks up iron in the baby's intestinal tract making it unavailable to harmful bacteria which need iron to survive.

LIBIDO: Sexual drive.

LIPIDS: Any of a large group of organic compounds, which are oily to the touch and insoluble in water. Lipids are a source of stored energy and are a component of cell membranes.

LACTOGENESIS: The phase during which milk production and secretion is established. Lactogenesis occurs in three stages: initiation of milk synthesis, copious milk production, and the establishment of mature milk supply.

Let-down Reflex: Also known as Milk Ejection Reflex, it is the spontaneous milk ejection from the breast triggered by external stimuli. It is often accompanied by a tingling sensation.

Luteal Phase: All days of elevated basal body temperatures following ovulation up to the first day of menstruation in the next cycle.

Mammary Organ: The breast functions as an organ when it extracts materials from the blood and converts them into milk.

Mastitis: Inflammation of the breast, also known as a breast infection.

Mature milk: Composition of human milk after seven to ten days postpartum.

Mechanical Breastfeeding Issues: When mother's milk is inefficiently or ineffectively transferred from breast to baby.

Menses: Periodic flow of blood from the uterus after ovulation.

Milk Ejection Reflex: See Let-down Reflex.

Mixed Breastfeeding: Formula or pumped breast milk given in addition to breastfeeding prior to a baby's sixth month.

Natural Family Planning: A means of reading a woman's signs of fertility and infertility; also known as fertility awareness.

Occlusion: The bringing of the opposing surfaces of the teeth (jaws) into contact.

Over-the-Counter Medications: Medications that can be obtained without a prescription. A common abbreviation for them is OTC.

Ovulation: Release of the female ovum or egg from the ovary.

Oxidative Stress: A stress to the defense system of an infant.

Oxytocin: A breastfeeding hormone produced in the pituitary gland. It is released during nipple stimulation causing the milk ejection reflex and uterine contractions.

Palate: The hard and soft portions of the roof of the mouth.

Placenta: Spongy structure that grows on the wall of the uterus during pregnancy and by which a baby is nourished during gestation.

Prescription Drugs and Medicines: Medications obtained from a pharmacy once a patient has been given a written order from a physician.

PRONE: Lying on one's stomach.

PITUITARY-OVARIAN AXIS: A two-way communication system between the brain and the ovaries, which coordinates the timing of ovulation, the production of hormones, and either the maintenance of a pregnancy or the onset of a menstrual period.

POSTPARTUM: Normally defined as the six week period following childbirth. In this text, the term also means the period after a childbirth experience.

PRETERM INFANT: An infant born before thirty-seven weeks gestation. Premature infant, or preemie, are terms also commonly used.

PROLACTIN: A hormone produced in the pituitary gland that stimulates the development of the breast and controls milk syntheses. Non pregnant levels in women are normally within the range of 10-25ng/dl compared to 200-400ng/dl for postpartum mothers.

PARADOX: Contradictions or opposite positions.

SECRETORY IgA: One of the most common antibodies found in all secretions of the body. IgA combines with proteins in the mucosa and defends body surfaces against invading micro-organisms.

SUPINE: Lying flat on one's back.

SUPPLEMENTARY FEEDING: Feedings that begin to replace breastfeeding calories; as a result breastfeeding frequency and intensity decreases gradually as feedings change from complementary to supplementary feeding. This leads to the eventual weaning from the breast although breastfeeding can still occur.

WEANING: Cessation of breastfeeding influenced either by mother, baby or both.

Index

C

G

H

I